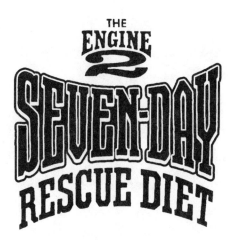

Also by Rip Esselstyn

The Engine 2 Diet: The Texas Firefighter's 28-Day Save-Your-Life Plan that Lowers Cholesterol and Burns Away the Pounds

Plant-Strong: Discover the World's Healthiest Diet

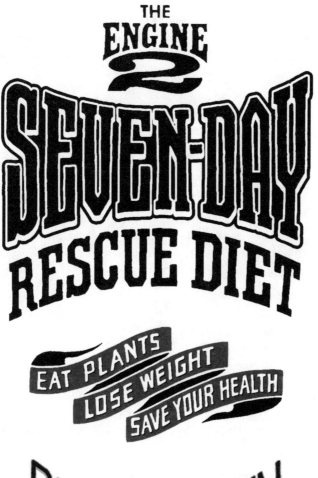

THE ENGINE 2 SEVEN-DAY RESCUE DIET

EAT PLANTS · LOSE WEIGHT · SAVE YOUR HEALTH

RIP ESSELSTYN

With recipes by Jane Esselstyn

GRAND CENTRAL
Life & Style

NEW YORK · BOSTON

Copyright © 2016 by Rip Esselstyn
Cover design and hand lettering by Jon Contino. Cover copyright © 2016 by Hachette Book Group, Inc.

Grand Central Life & Style
Hachette Book Group
1290 Avenue of the Americas, New York, NY 10104
grandcentrallifeandstyle.com
twitter.com/grandcentralpub

First Edition: December 2016

Grand Central Life & Style is an imprint of Grand Central Publishing. The Grand Central Life & Style name and logo are trademarks of Hachette Book Group, Inc.

The publisher is not responsible for websites (or their content) that are not owned by the publisher.

The Hachette Speakers Bureau provides a wide range of authors for speaking events. To find out more, go to www.hachettespeakersbureau.com or call (866) 376-6591.

Library of Congress Cataloging-in-Publication Data has been applied for.

ISBNs: 978-1-4555-9117-6 (hardcover); 978-1-4555-9115-2 (ebook)

Printed in the United States of America

LSC-H

10 9 8 7 6 5 4 3 2 1

For our children: Kole, Sophie, and Hope. You light up our world.

Dear Reader:

I'm Rip Esselstyn and I want to thank you for picking up *The Engine 2 Seven-Day Rescue Diet*. If you follow the seven simple principles in this book, you will lose weight, lower your cholesterol, and feel great! All of this in just seven short, delicious days.

What are the seven principles I want you to follow for seven days?

- Eat plants.
- Eat whole foods.
- Chew your calories.
- Avoid calorie-dense foods.
- Limit your protein.
- Limit your salt, sugar, and fat.
- Walk every day.

That's it! No problem, right?

Now, to guarantee you have a successful week, the second half of the book is filled with easy and delicious recipes. I've also included charts that show you how to build amazingly healthy bowls for every meal of the day. These bowls are fun, calorie light, nutrient dense, and filled with fiber. They are downright bowlicious!

This book is based on the staggering results that more than 1,200 people achieved at the seven-day immersion programs I've run over the last six years. Now you can achieve these same results at home! Show yourself that what you thought was impossible is totally possible. And when you're ready to celebrate, share your results at info@engine2.com and we'll give you a "Kale Yeah!" shout-out.

Eat plant-strong!

Rip

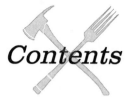

Contents

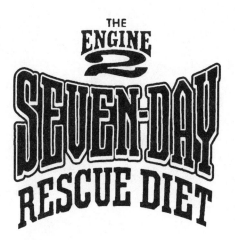

Introduction

The week of December 13, 2004, began on a cold and rainy Monday in Austin, Texas. It was the start of some torturous days, but such moments are not uncommon for a firefighter.

Our first call came in to the Engine 2 station at 5:00 a.m.: "Lifting assistance." This meant that EMS needed us to help them lift and carry a patient into the ambulance. Unfortunately, this wasn't unusual. This call was like so many others in which we had to help EMS carry people who were morbidly obese. This time, it was a forty-four-year-old woman who weighed 450 pounds and couldn't walk; plus, the hallways in her home were so narrow and abrupt that the stretcher wouldn't fit. We lifted her onto a thick wool blanket, and then we had to maneuver her around tight corners and down the stairway. (Today, instead of blankets, fire departments use a "MegaMover," a compact, portable piece of durable material with fourteen handles that can hold up to 1,000 pounds, which was created specifically for the onslaught of lifting-assistance calls that fire and EMS workers respond to.)

It took eight of us to accomplish the task. We positioned two people on each side of the blanket, two people at the front of the blanket, and two people at the rear of the blanket, while one person guided us down the stairs from the front and the eighth person guided us from the rear. Down we went, one step at a time, until we reached the front door, at which point we moved the patient from the blanket onto a hydraulic stretcher and then into the ambulance. (Hydraulic stretchers can handle up to 500 pounds and take a tremendous burden off the backs of emergency service workers—we were throwing out our backs left and right before their existence.)

After we loaded the woman into the ambulance, I asked the EMS workers why she was being transported to the hospital. They told me she had a fever from an infection in her lower leg that wasn't healing and they needed the doctors to look at it. Along with being overweight, the woman had type 2 diabetes. Obesity is actually one of the biggest risk factors for diabetes, which is why the latest term for this one-two punch of obesity with diabetes is "diobesity." It is becoming an epidemic in North America.

Back to the station we went. As often happens, we weren't there long. We had many other calls involving medical issues that day, including a young man reported as either asleep or unconscious in his car. We slid down the pole—yes, Engine 2 is one of only two stations in Austin that still have a real firefighter's pole—and took off. When we arrived we found the patient shaking uncontrollably, freezing cold, and sweating profusely.

Glancing at his wrist, we noticed a bracelet that indicated he was diabetic. The very first thing we did was check the man's blood sugar. It was a paltry 19 mg/dl (milligrams per deciliter). Anything under 50 mg/dl is considered low. Nineteen mg/dl is dangerously low. When a diabetic patient is unconscious, you can't give him glucose orally, so we waited for EMS to arrive. When they did, they immediately set up an IV and gave the man a shot of glucose. In less than a minute he shot upright and asked, "What the hell is going on?"

We told him his blood sugar had fallen down to 19. He replied that he couldn't believe it. He had felt tired, decided to take a nap, and that was the last thing he remembered. He said he had been diagnosed as a type 2 diabetic four years previously, at age fifteen. Fifteen! We gave him some solid food to help keep his blood sugar levels elevated for a sustained period and told him to be really careful in the future—this was a matter of life and death.

Another typical call that week came from one of the University of Texas dorm rooms, where an eighteen-year-old female was suffering from generalized sickness. As is routine, we took her medical history, whereupon she told us that on the advice of her family physician, she was taking 10 mg (milligrams) of Lipitor daily to deal with her high cholesterol levels.

When EMS arrived, they cut us loose, but as we drove back to the station we all remarked on how crazy it was that someone so young could already be on the road to a lifetime of medications. If her doctor were truly effective, instead of being a glorified prescription writer, he or she would inform the patient of the benefits of eating well. The right diet can help avoid a cocktail of daily medications.

Later that same week, a call came in concerning an unconscious male at one of the University of Texas banquet halls. We arrived on the scene to find a forty-eight-year-old man, lying on his back on the ground, breathless and pulseless. We were told he had suddenly collapsed; as it turned out, he'd had a full-blown heart attack.

We immediately started chest compressions while two members of our crew got the AED (automatic external defibrillator) set up. We stopped chest compressions, placed the pads on the man's chest, and waited for what's called a shockable rhythm. This essentially gives rescue workers permission to shock a patient in hopes of restarting the heart. We attempted this two times without any luck, so we continued chest compressions until EMS arrived.

EMS intubated the patient, and then we worked in harmony to resuscitate him with a combination of shocks and compressions. After thirty minutes without success, EMS decided it was time to call the emergency room doctor and pronounce the patient dead. The sad reality is that every forty-three seconds someone has a heart attack; and every minute and twenty-three seconds someone in America dies from a massive heart attack. Over the course of my dozen years with the Austin Fire Department, we responded to more than fifty heart attacks and we were able to resuscitate only three patients.

We received more than a dozen medical calls during our shifts at the firehouse that week. It was a sobering week of medical calls, but we also had one chance to do what we joined the department to do—we fought a fire!

At 8:55 a.m. on a very cold Sunday, just as we were finishing breakfast, dispatch reported a house fire at an address 1.5 miles from our station. We jumped into the fire truck and immediately switched from medical mode to fire mode.

When we arrived, the house was almost completely engulfed in flames. We were the second engine company to arrive (Engine 3 got there first), so our job was to supply water to them from our 500-gallon tank and help deploy hose lines to fight the fire.

The flames were so high, and the wind so strong, that we had to put our truck in reverse and back up several hundred feet. As we did, the electrical wires in front of the house started arcing, the transformers exploded, and sparks flew everywhere. The smoke was so heavy it was almost impossible to see within a hundred-foot radius of the house.

Because the fire had grown increasingly dangerous in such a short time, the incident commander called a Mayday, which means that everyone must immediately get out of the building and move to a safe zone. He shifted operations from offensive to defensive mode as well, fighting the fire from outside the structure instead of from inside. He also called a second alarm, which resulted in two more fire engines and one more ladder company showing up—bringing more resources and more firefighter power.

The closest fire hydrant was inaccessible because of the immense heat and flames, so my co-firefighter Derick and I were asked to find another hydrant. We had to move more than 600 feet of 200-pound, 5-inch supply hose up a hill before we located one. While we were desperately pulling, Derick yelled at the onlookers to give us a hand; soon six good Samaritans were struggling along with us until we had access to an unlimited supply of water.

We did our best, but the fire was overwhelming. Engine 2 Company was now assigned the south sector of the fire and instructed to protect the adjacent house. We put several hose lines in place and shot tons of water onto the house to keep it from catching fire. Unfortunately, the heat and flames were so strong that one side of the two-story duplex adjacent to the burning house caught fire as well. Even road signs and cars parked on the street were melting; the emergency lights on Engine 3 melted—it was parked more than 100 feet away—and its windshield cracked.

After two hours the fire was finally put out by a group of tired, wet, and cold firefighters. We later learned it had all started with a cigarette. One lousy cigarette.

When I became a firefighter in 1997, I assumed that most of my job would entail fighting fires like that last one. Not even close! Most of what a firefighter does is take care of all the sick and ailing people who need help because they don't understand that their diets are causing their health to suffer.

Now let me tell you about another week, six years later. By that time I had left the Austin Fire Department following the blazing success of my first book, *The Engine 2 Diet*. The book documents my personal journey with a plant-based diet, as well as the medical science behind it, and tells how I got a bunch of Texas firefighters to eat nothing but plants all day. I had discovered a deep desire to help people and save lives and was bringing those efforts to a whole new level by becoming a full-time crusader for plant-based foods. I began throwing Engine 2 events around the country. I wrote another book about the benefits of eating plant-strong foods. (I came up with the term "plant-strong" because plants truly are the strongest and healthiest foods on the planet.) I gave talks and seminars to thousands of people a year. And, I began an exciting relationship with Whole Foods Market as one of its healthy-eating partners in conjunction with developing a line of superhealthy Engine 2 food products.

As part of my partnership with Whole Foods Market, I started holding retreats for their unhealthiest employees (they had to medically qualify to attend), with Whole Foods picking up the tab. The company's CEO, John Mackey, who understands that a plant-based diet can prevent and reverse chronic disease, decided to allocate millions of dollars annually to educate his employees with this gift of health. The retreat programs were at first exclusively for Whole Foods Market employees, but after two years we broadened the program, opening it up to members of the public as well. For one week, these participants live and breathe the plant-strong lifestyle. They eat a delicious array of whole-food, plant-based meals. They enjoy morning exercises and afternoon hikes. They soak up entertaining and educational lectures given by the best plant-based minds in the world. They literally eat up the cooking demonstrations, and they bask in daily interactive applied-learning exercises with the other participants. Add all this up and it's a powerful formula that enables people to rescue their health. They now hold the keys to preventing and reversing the worst of the chronic Western killer diseases.

During one of these weeklong rescues, I met David Honoré, a forty-eight-year-old native of Philadelphia, who, like most of us, grew up eating the standard American diet, which is rooted in meat, dairy, and processed foods. But David didn't just eat meat daily. He ate it several times a day. And he loved it! "I was the king of meat," he admitted. "I ate enough for three lifetimes!"

However, David's body didn't love meat, nor did it love the other processed foods, fat, and dairy he was consuming. By the time he reached forty, David had developed several serious health issues, including type

2 diabetes and high blood pressure, and he was having challenges "raising the flag." To remedy all this, he was taking eight different prescription medicines and was a candidate for even more.

It never occurred to David that his bad health might have been a result of his diet—that is, until he spotted a memo at work about an Engine 2 Rescue program. The memo explained the relationship between diet, exercise, and health and promised that the program could help restore well-being. After taking a good, hard look at himself, David realized that he was on a self-proclaimed "collision course with destruction."

He applied and was accepted into the program, and a few months later he flew off to Sedona, Arizona. His last animal-based meal was an oversize pork breakfast sausage at the airport.

David arrived in Sedona scared of what the program might ask him to do, and he was worried that he wouldn't like the food. Instead, he loved everything he ate and enjoyed the program immensely. Best of all, in just seven days David cut his total cholesterol level in half! It had been as high as 280 mg/dl, but his doctor had put him on statins, bringing it down to 180 mg/dl when he arrived in Arizona. By the end of the week, it had dropped all the way down to 95 mg/dl.

Not only that, but David's blood pressure improved, dropping from 142/83 to 134/74. His triglycerides fell from 133 mg/dl to 71 mg/dl, and his LDL ("bad") cholesterol plummeted from 112 mg/dl to 53 mg/dl. As a bonus, he dropped 8 pounds without even trying.

All in seven days!

David decided that if he could achieve these benefits in just one week, what could he accomplish if he gave it a year? So he did. As of today, he has lost another 70 pounds and is off every one of his medications. Best of all, his diabetes has disappeared.

David says he feels like a new person. He has energy again. His skin is no longer puffy. For the first time in as long as he can remember, his feet—which had become swollen and disfigured because of his diabetes—are now as attractive and svelte as the rest of his body, and he proudly parades around in flip-flops! Once a part-time opera singer, David found that his amazing tenor voice, which had been failing, returned, allowing him to perform with all the gusto of old. Furthermore, he enjoys food more than ever because his taste buds have come alive. He has even taken up running—he learned that exercise can be enjoyable and is the cherry that tops off the plant-strong lifestyle!

Sadly, two months after David returned from the Engine 2 Rescue program, his mother died after falling into a diabetic coma. He wants to make sure he stays alive to see his ten-year-old daughter grow up to marry and have children. Most important, he wants to leave a legacy of health for the next generation of Honorés. And for the first time, he feels confident that he will.

All of this happened in seven spectacularly wonderful days. And it wasn't just David who had such an inspiring story to tell. What made this week so wonderful was that almost all of the other 90 people in David's group had similar, spectacular results! That's what happens when people start taking care of themselves and shift their diet to powerful healing plants. They no longer have to call the fire department for help. They are able to rescue their own health.

> This was a life-changing experience for me. Before Rip's program, eating plant-based seemed like one of those difficult "out of my league" kind of lifestyles. Now it is a simple no-brainer. Who wouldn't want to eat gorgeous, delicious food that is easy to prepare and makes you feel wonderful?!
>
> —Lisa Hamilton, age 61, retired RN

Myself, I have been living the plant-strong lifestyle for more than thirty years now. In that time I've been a world-class triathlete, a firefighter in the Austin, Texas, fire department, a husband, a father of three children, and a healthy-eating partner for Whole Foods Market. I have also written two best-selling books on the subject of plant-based nutrition—*The Engine 2 Diet* and *Plant-Strong* (originally published as *My Beef with Meat*)—and I have toured all over the world sharing this message of health and hope: that a plant-savvy diet is the best way to protect yourself from the onslaught of chronic Western diseases (which you will read more about in chapter 1).

Engine 2 started with a firehouse bet to see who had the lowest cholesterol level. This single bet inspired my fellow firefighters to eat a bunch of plants and motivated me to write *The Engine 2 Diet*. The research for the book and the book itself ignited a healthy-eating revolution within the Austin Fire Department that sent ripples throughout the country.

My knowledge of eating a plant-based diet came from my father (and my hero), Dr. Caldwell B. Esselstyn Jr., who, besides winning a gold medal in the 1956 Olympics for rowing, was one of the Cleveland Clinic's top surgeons, president of the clinic's medical staff, and chairman of its Breast Cancer Task Force. (The clinic was actually founded in 1921 by my maternal great-grandfather, George Crile Sr.) In 1985, after many years of being stymied by treating disease with conventional medicine, my father took a decidedly new approach: convinced that nutrition played an important role in health, he asked the clinic's cardiology department to send him patients coping with serious heart disease—among them they had suffered forty-nine coronary events over the previous eight years—and he placed them on a plant-based diet. A dozen years later all but one of the patients was heart-healthy! The only one who wasn't had strayed from the diet. For obvious reasons, my entire family then became plant-based eaters.

To back up the claims behind my first book, I decided to conduct my own study. I asked the participants to eat nothing but terrific, delicious plant-based foods for six weeks. Everyone who followed the program had amazing results. They lost weight, their cholesterol levels dropped, and they felt terrific. I arranged a second study, but this time reduced it from six to four weeks, and discovered that we could get equally excellent results in twenty-eight days—and thus the program for *The Engine 2 Diet: The Texas Firefighter's 28-Day Plan that Lowers Cholesterol and Burns Away the Pounds* was born. My second book gave newly converted plant-based eaters a guide to answer every question they could ever ask about eating plants—and once again I toured the world sharing the message.

Along the way, in between all that touring and traveling and experimentation, I learned something that I could never have guessed when I started my initial studies back in 2007. I had assumed that twenty-eight days was the absolute minimum time necessary to see results. Boy, was I wrong! In 2008 I asked four of the firefighters at Station 4 to take the twenty-eight-day challenge. They said that twenty-eight days was just too long and wasn't going to "butter the biscuit"; however, they'd be willing to give me fourteen days. The results? After fourteen days they had all dropped their weight, cholesterol, and triglyceride levels substantially. At that point I knew the body could make profound internal changes in as little as two weeks. But I still never imagined anyone could budge their cholesterol, LDL, and blood pressure in less time.

Again, I was wrong. I learned just how wrong when I started hosting many more Engine 2 Seven-Day Rescue programs, programs that have given more than 1,000 people the opportunity to improve their health, expand their minds, and activate their taste buds to levels they never dreamed possible. A quick look at the average drop in our participants' standard biometric markers over six years of throwing these seven-day retreats shows the breathtaking way the body can begin to heal and get healthy in *just one week*!

Engine 2 Rescue Program Average Results

Cholesterol	−26 mg/dl
LDL cholesterol	−24 mg/dl
Triglycerides	−23 mg/dl
Blood pressure	−10/5 mm/Hg
Weight	−3.0 lbs.

Think about that. Seven days. That's 168 hours out of your waking life. Just 168 hours, and your life will change forever! I didn't believe it could happen until I started seeing it work in my Seven-Day Rescue programs, again and again, and with all kinds of people from all kinds of backgrounds.

I started hosting these Seven-Day Rescue programs in 2010. By 2017 we had completed eleven of them. And they were all successful. Of course, it's a dream when you can check out from reality for seven days in the mountains and you don't have to cook a meal, make a bed, wash a dish, or drive a car—where your only responsibility is to take care of yourself, soak up the information, eat delicious plant-strong foods, and bond with your fellow participants. But not everyone can take a week off from work and join me in the mountains of Sedona, so I decided I needed to test the merits of the program in the real world with people who were living real lives with real jobs.

Let me tell you about one pilot study in particular, because it's the most recent. This study took place when I partnered with an Ohio group called North Ridgeville Heart and Sole, which was working to decrease the rate of cardiovascular disease and chronic illness in its community through many different initiatives, and the group volunteered to help organize a pilot study for this book.

In October 2015, we placed an ad in the local paper looking for participants willing to test-drive the Engine 2 Diet for seven days. We also recruited North Ridgeville city leadership to join in this grant-funded experiment. We quickly found that the promise of real, measured results in just one week made even the most resistant skeptics eager to join. Within two days we had 60 people ready to start their seven-day journey and a waiting list of more than 100 more.

Participants included citizens from all walks of life in the community: teachers, lawyers, businessmen, school principals, firefighters, cops, students, and even the North Ridgeville mayor and his wife. The group was 36 percent male and 64 percent female, ranging in age from sixteen to seventy-one, with an average age of fifty-one.

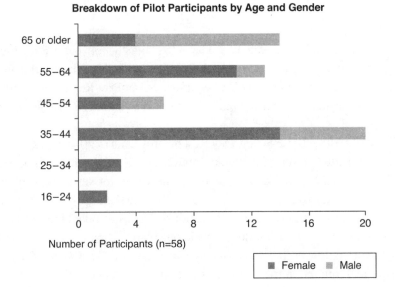

Breakdown of Pilot Participants by Age and Gender

All of the participants were required to take before-and-after biometric screenings so we could document their results, test the efficacy of the program, and collect the data for this book. We weighed them and took their blood pressure. We partnered with a laboratory and hired several phlebotomists to draw blood so we could test for total cholesterol, LDL cholesterol, HDL cholesterol, triglycerides, and fasting blood sugar.

Every participant received an eighty-page booklet that contained an overview of the "Rescue," along with the same meal plans and recipe concepts you have in this book. They also committed to keeping a daily food log that they would e-mail at the end of every day to one of the Engine 2 Rescue program coaches. We found this to be imperative to people's success from an accountability standpoint, as well as giving the Engine 2 coaches the opportunity to offer guidance, feedback, course corrections, and encouragement.

At the end of the seven days we asked all the participants to show up at a centralized location after fasting for twelve hours for their post biometric screenings. Then we weighed them, took their blood pressures, and drew their blood just as we had done the previous week.

The results were more than consistent with the other studies we've done. In fact, I was flat out over the moon with the results!

> **Weight:** One hundred percent of the participants lost weight. The average weight loss per participant was 6 pounds; the maximum weight loss was 14 pounds. For details on the participants' weight loss, please refer to the chart below.
>
> **Total Cholesterol:** Ninety-five percent of participants dropped their total cholesterol levels. The average drop was 32 mg/dl, with a maximum drop of 76 points. Seventy-five percent

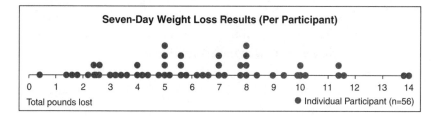

of participants dropped their total cholesterol between 21 and 76 points.

LDL Cholesterol: Eighty-nine percent of participants dropped their LDL—or lethal, as I call it—cholesterol. The average drop was 22 mg/dl. The maximum drop was 50 points.

HDL Cholesterol: Eighty-eight percent of participants dropped their HDL—the "good"—cholesterol. The average drop was 9 mg/dl. The maximum drop was 34 points. Now, it is true that HDL cholesterol is associated with a decreased risk of heart disease, and some people and their doctors are concerned when their HDL levels decline. However, lowering HDL cholesterol when you lower total cholesterol is normal and a good thing. As your total cholesterol drops, both its HDL and LDL components drop as well. This is because as you clean up your internal chemistry, your body doesn't make as many of the HDL mopper-upper cholesterols. There's no need for them anymore! And the ones you keep become bigger, more efficient mopper-uppers. For more details on changes in cholesterol levels, refer to the charts in Appendix 3.

Blood Pressure: Sixty-seven percent of the group dropped their blood pressure. The average drop in systolic pressure (the upper number) was 15 points, with 25 percent of participants reducing it by 18 to 49 points. The average drop in diastolic pressure (the lower number) was 10 points, with 25 percent reducing it by 12 to 29 points.

Triglycerides: Sixty percent dropped their triglycerides, with 25 percent reducing them by 82 to 358 points. The average triglyceride reduction was 75 points. The maximum reduction was 1,438 points.

Fasting Blood Sugar: Twenty-three people started the week with a fasting blood sugar over 100 mg/dl, indicating they were prediabetic or diabetic. Of those 23, 8 dropped their blood sugar below 100mg/dl by the end of the week, indicating they were now in the "normal" range.

(For a complete analysis of the North Ridgeville Study, see page 283.)

The truth is, I observed statistically significant improvements in all biometric measures in our pilot group: total cholesterol, LDL, HDL, glucose, triglycerides, systolic and diastolic blood pressures, and weight. Moreover, nearly three-quarters of respondents said that they would remain fully plant-strong or remain plant-strong most of the time.

Now, many physicians would tell you these results are too good to be true and that only an error from the laboratory—or a miracle—could possibly explain them. However, we know better. People who adhere to this Rescue program for the full seven days get these incredible results 100 percent of the time.

Participant after participant remarked after getting back their blood work, losing weight, and dropping their blood pressure: "I'm sold!"; "Oh my god, this really works!"; "Somebody pinch me!"; and "It's a miracle!" No, actually it is not a miracle. There are no sleight-of-hand or cheap parlor tricks involved. It's just good old-fashioned strong-food nutrition. The most underused and overlooked tool in the medicine cabinet or on a doctor's prescription pad is the food at the end of your fork.

I was excited to try Rip's program, especially since it was only seven days. As each day went by I could feel the difference in the way my body was reacting to the process, and I could SEE the difference in the way my clothes fit. The end results I received via my wellness screening solidified what I already knew: This program showed me more in seven days than some other diets can show in three months. This is not a diet…it is a life changer, and I will definitely incorporate it more into my daily life.
—Heidi Bayer, age 41, executive assistant

I want you to experience the same life-changing results as our Engine 2 Seven-Day Rescue participants did. I want you to go just seven days without eating any animal protein, animal flesh, or animal by-products. You won't be eating any processed and refined carbohydrates, either.

No trashy calories that are a nutritional black hole. You also won't be eating a lot of calorie-rich, high-fat foods like avocados and nuts, nor any processed oils. You'll just be eating the best and strongest foods in the world and getting the biggest bang for your calorie buck.

Here's what I promise you: not only will you feel better than you have in years, you'll lose weight (typical results are between 3 and 14 pounds), your total cholesterol level will be much more attractive, your LDL cholesterol will no longer be lethal, your triglycerides will be on the downslide, your energy will be on the upswing, and your poops will be easy and on schedule.

You'll be on a path to a life free of medications. Statins, blood pressure medications, and diabetes drugs address the symptoms of these diseases, but they do nothing to address the underlying cause: the food. Just as the slew of chronic Western diseases are the manifestations of our unhealthy food choices day after day, week after week, and year after year, you will see the opposite when you make healthy food choices each day. And after you've strung together just seven of these days, your body starts to rapidly detox and remove unwanted cholesterol, inflammation, body fat, and a bunch of other debris that has accumulated at a molecular and cellular level in your body for decades.

You'll also discover all kinds of wonderful foods you may never have eaten before—and you'll find that these foods will fill you up, taste great, and keep your whole body healthy.

Before you start, I absolutely, 100 percent insist you devour the seven chapters that precede the recipe section. This is the core information that is crucial in helping you understand the ins and outs of the program and how the Engine 2 Rescue will work for you. Some of this information is similar to what I've written about before, such as the benefits of a plant-based diet to your health, but much of it is based on seminal research that has come to light only in the last few years. One of the most rewarding parts of being a crusader for this kind of eating is that medical science is constantly publishing more and more proof that there's no healthier way to eat than a plant-based diet. It seems that almost every week a new study appears that validates everything my father and I have been saying for years!

In the second part of the book we'll get down to the brass tacks of the seven-day program. You will love how easy it is. You will light up like a carved pumpkin at Halloween when you taste how delicious the food is. And to prove it, you will find dozens of recipes to keep you happy and full for the entire week—dishes that can be prepared by people for whom the kitchen is a distant and foreign location, as well as by people for whom cooking is the greatest joy in life. There's something here for everyone.

So get ready to have the most wonderful, mouthwatering seven-day adventure of your life. Make it happen!

My husband signed me up and said "Let's do this!" He was less than excited as he is a huge meat eater, but he and I both stayed true all week long. At the end of the week I was amazed at how much better I felt. My arthritis pain has greatly diminished, the swelling in my feet and legs has improved, and I have more energy than I have had in years! Overall I feel better than I have in a very long time. Is eating a cheeseburger more important than that?

—Beverly Gillock, age 66, retired
board of elections coordinator

PART I

1

Why We Love Plants

Back in 2005 the *Austin American-Statesman* ran an article called "Tofu Outmuscles Red Meat at Firehouse." At the time I was helping my fellow firefighters at the Engine 2 firehouse become fire-breathing, dragon-slaying, plant-based demigods. That tofu comment made for a catchy headline, and the article made our firehouse famous, but it's more than catchy. It's true. Tofu does outmuscle red meat.

Actually, to be fair, it's not just tofu. All plant foods outmuscle all animal foods. Whether you're eating legumes like hummus and tofu, fruits like oranges and strawberries, vegetables like broccoli and potatoes, or whole grains like oatmeal and brown rice, plants can out-tackle, outperform, and outlast any hunk of meat, eggs, or dairy you throw at them.

That's right. When it comes to health- and performance-promoting nutrients per calorie, there's no contest. There is no greater bang for your calorie buck than the kick you get from plants. Plants cross the finish line while meat is wheezing and gasping at the halfway mark.

In spite of all the scientific evidence that proves the power of plants—and I will get into that later—there's a misconception out there that meat is somehow manly while plants are weak and timid. That's strange. Aside from those "Rocky Mountain oysters" you hear about, I'd never concede that you might be eating a "manly" food when you're eating an animal product.

In fact, in this book you're going to hear the term "strong food" often. What does that mean, exactly? Hint: strong foods have nothing to do with meat or dairy or those junky "muscle milk" powders and snack bars that purport to make you stronger.

Here's the short answer: Plants are strong foods. Animal products are weak foods.

Wait, does that sound right? Aren't big, juicy T-bone steaks strong food? If you ever travel across my home state of Texas, you're likely to see a wide range of steak houses, including one that even offers this challenge: finish a 72-ounce steak in an hour and your photo goes up on the wall and your meal is on the house. (Unfortunately, your future medical bills aren't.) You might think some of these champs are healthy sorts, but in reality all that meat is rotting them away from the inside. If people really understood what makes a food strong, you might be seeing spinach-eating contests instead.

So what is it that makes a food strong?

I'm a 160-pound man. I exercised regularly and ate pretty well, yet my cholesterol was still borderline to high for the past three years of biometric readings. I stuck to Rip's diet for seven days and I dropped 25 points off of my total cholesterol. I have completely eliminated the thought that high cholesterol is hereditary for me!

—Brandon Chesla, age 62, technical analyst

Strong and Healthy Macronutrients

Macronutrients are some of the most important nutrients you eat. The word *macro* means "large," and, sure enough, you need a large amount of macronutrients for your growth, metabolism, and all your other basic life functions.

The three primary macronutrients are pretty well known: carbohydrates, fat, and protein. You need all three to live, no exceptions. So it makes sense that the food you eat should have all three, right?

Animal meat contains only two macronutrients: fat and protein. They're missing the number one source of fuel for your body: carbohydrates. On the other hand, healthy and unprocessed carbohydrates make up anywhere from 20 to 80 percent of the calories in fruits, vegetables, whole grains, and legumes, leaving you with a slow and steady release of energy. Ask any endurance athlete what he or she loads up on before a big race. It's not eggs and steak. It's carbs. Lots of carbs.

During digestion, your body breaks down carbs into glucose, which enters your bloodstream and provides energy to your cells. The more healthy unprocessed carbs you eat, the more energy you have.

How about fat? It's true that animal products do have lots of fat, and some fat is necessary in the human diet. But not all fat is created equal. Fats have a light side and a dark side. The Luke Skywalker fats you find in plants—healthy, essential omega-3 and omega-6 fats—are associated with a reduced risk of heart disease, diabetes, breast cancer, and colon cancer among many other chronic diseases. By eating a simple plant-strong diet, you get all the essential fats you need without any of the unnecessary and disease-promoting ones—in other words, the fats you find in meat and dairy products.

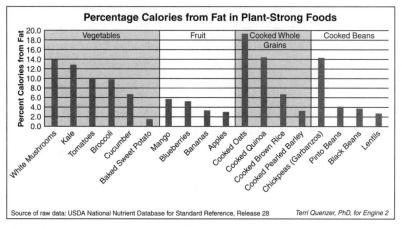

Here's the real skinny on fats in plants!

I call these dark-side fats—the evil Darth Vader fats of the trans and saturated varieties. Both occur naturally in meat and dairy (and can be found in processed junk food). If you eat too many of these dark-side fats, you'll end up breathing just like Darth himself. That's because saturated fats and trans fats cause plaque-promoting inflammation in your arteries, which leads to heart disease, and also encourages insulin resistance in your muscle cells, which leads to diabetes. Moreover, the

Harvard Women's Health Study, which has been following thousands of women for more than two decades, found that women with the highest saturated-fat intake had a 60 to 70 percent greater chance of experiencing cognitive decline.

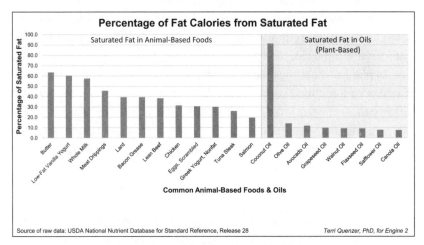

There are artery-clogging saturated fats in all animal products and even processed oils. Save your arteries and steer clear of this unnecessary weak fat!

Whether it's a bird with wings, a cow with hooves, a fish with fins, or an egg in a shell, saturated and trans fats are lurking in every animal product you eat. If you eat animals, you can't escape these fats. By choosing plants, however, you can rest (and eat) assured that you are taking in all the strong fats you need without any of the weak, disease-promoting ones.

Trans Fats

By now you've probably heard about the dangers of trans fats. These are fats that manufacturers induce in foods during the process of partial hydrogenation in which hydrogen gas is bubbled through vegetable oil. This process increases the product's shelf life. Trans fats raise your LDL (bad) cholesterol and lower your HDL (good) cholesterol. But many people think they're safe from the dangers of trans fat. After all, there have been numerous highly publicized trans-fat bans in cities like New York and San Francisco, and food labels almost universally boast "0 grams of trans fat" even on the most suspect products.

Be careful. There are lots of loopholes food manufacturers use to fool you. If a food has less than 0.5 gram of trans fat per serving, the manufacturer is allowed to pretend the product doesn't have any trans fat at all. Be sure to check the ingredients list as well. Look for partially hydrogenated oils, a telltale sign that you're eating trans fats. If you aren't careful, the amount of trans fat you eat on a daily basis can add up quickly. To be clear, there is no safe amount of trans fat.

Why not err on the side of caution and choose mostly foods without any labels at all: fruits and veggies?

The third macronutrient is protein. We'll talk about this more in chapter 5, but there are two huge misconceptions out there about protein. The first is that you need a great deal of it to be healthy and strong. The second is that you can't get enough of it from plants. Both are wrong.

The truth is, according to the World Health Organization, at most 10 to 15 percent of your calories need to come from protein. Why not get it all from plants? Plant-based proteins contain all eight of the essential amino acids, and all in the right balance. Animal protein, however, throws this delicate balance into complete disarray. These weak proteins cannibalize calcium from your bones, which contributes to osteoporosis, not to mention accelerating the growth of cancers by boosting levels of the cancer-causing hormone IGF-1 (insulin-like growth factor).

Animal protein is not just weak food—it's toxic food. Highly acidic animal proteins inundate your kidneys with acid, causing them to enter a frenzied state called hyperfiltration. Imagine constantly revving your car engine at the red line. It wouldn't last long, right? The same goes for your kidneys. By continually forcing them to filter out all the animal junk from your blood, they get weaker and weaker and, eventually, may fail. Why else do you think that a Johns Hopkins University study concluded that as few as 41 percent of Americans have normal kidney function, or that Tufts Medical Center researchers believe that one in three people over the age of sixty-four may be suffering from chronic kidney disease?

Plant protein, on the other hand, has been shown to protect healthy kidneys as well as help sick kidneys become better by easing their burden.

Eat Like Tom and Gisele

Ever wondered how Tom Brady, the most clutch NFL quarterback of all time, and his wife, Gisele Bündchen, the most successful supermodel of all time, eat in their own home?

Meet Allen Campbell, the Brady family's personal chef. Allen is a graduate of T. Colin Campbell's plant-based nutrition course at Cornell University. "My philosophy is that a plant-based diet has the power to reverse and prevent disease," Allen told Boston.com in an interview. "I had started really focusing on plant-based diets, because that's where all the nutrition is." That's why 80 percent of what Allen cooks for Tom, Gisele, and their kids is fresh vegetables and whole grains. No added sugars, no sugary drinks, no dairy.

If you're aiming to play like Tom and shine like Gisele, you can't go wrong by starting with a whole food, plant-based diet!

Strong and Healthy Micronutrients

Carbohydrates, fat, and protein aren't the only nutrients. Micronu-trients such as vitamins and minerals are also essential to your health, development, and growth. Eleven out of the thirteen vitamins are found in plants (vitamin D comes from the sun, and vitamin B_{12} comes from microorganisms in the soil).

All seventeen of the major and minor essential minerals are found in plants. That's because plants romp and play in the soil all day long. Their best friends are minerals, which deposit themselves in plant roots, stems, and leaves. When you eat plants, whether it's broccoli, kale, or beans, you're getting pure, essential minerals straight from the source and in a highly absorbable form.

Did you know that the best source of retainable calcium comes from plants, not from milk? That's because the strong calcium found in greens, such as broccoli and kale, is absorbed into your blood twice as effectively as the calcium in dairy. Contrary to what dairy industry lobbyists might want you to believe, calcium does not actually come from cows. It originates from the soil, which a cow takes in from eating grass. In business, you try to cut out as many middlemen as possible to maximize profit. Why not cut out the middle-cow and maximize your health? There's more calcium in 4 ounces of fortified tofu, or ¾ cup of cooked collard greens, than in a whole glass of milk. Just 2 cups of good old-fashioned black beans contain 90 mg of calcium.

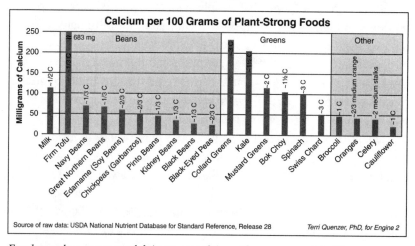

For those who say you need dairy to get calcium, I have one word: bull!

Meanwhile, some of the most exciting new research pertains to a special type of micronutrients called phytonutrients. These naturally occurring nutrients are found exclusively in plants and offer extraordinary health benefits.

For example, certain phytonutrients have been found to boost your defenses against pathogens and pollutants, increase blood flow (everywhere!), slow down the aging process, increase energy, decrease the number and size of cancerous polyps in the colon, and help prevent the formation of new blood vessels that feed cancerous tumors elsewhere in the body.

> I have had a lot of stomach problems, high cholesterol, and I am overweight. Since day one of the Seven-Day Rescue Diet, my stomach has not bothered me, [and] I have lost 8 pounds. I have actually enjoyed eating this way much more than I expected!
> —James McVeigh, age 68, retired city treasurer, North Ridgeville, Ohio

Furthermore, a 2013 nationwide survey by National Institutes of Health researchers found that people with the most carotenoid phytonutrients in their bloodstreams—the kind you find in tomatoes, sweet potatoes, and dark green leafy veggies, for instance—have a lower risk of depression. Indeed, a 2013 study published by the *Journal of Affective Disorders* involving a thousand elderly men and women found that those who ate tomatoes daily were half as likely to be depressed as those who ate tomatoes only once a week or less.

Scientists have so far discovered more than twenty thousand separate phytochemicals, and we're only just beginning to understand how special these plant nutrients are. Plants can't run away from their enemies, throw a punch, or bite and scratch, so they have to come up with other ways to protect themselves from invaders and predators. This is where phytonutrients come into the picture. Plants naturally make these amazing substances to ward off environmental hazards along with bugs and animals. They deploy a plethora of phytonutrients, and you benefit directly by consuming these strong little superheroes. They immediately go to work to fight disease, slow down the aging process, neutralize free radicals, and mitigate environmental oxidative stress.

A Strong and Healthy Environment

Plants don't just help your body—they help Mother Earth, too. Let's start with water. Take California, for instance, which is suffering a period of severe drought and is taking measures to conserve water. People can and should be mindful of water use, of course, but the media seem hell-bent on blaming fruits and vegetables. Poor, innocent little almonds in particular have come under fire for supposedly soaking up everyone's water. The devil's nut! How dare they! Eighty percent of California's water goes to agriculture, they say, so you should stop eating so much produce.

Actually, you should do the opposite. Yes, it's true that 80 percent of California's water is used for agriculture, but let's think about what—or rather who—is using all that water. People stop buying almonds because they think that product is contributing to California's water shortage, but what they should do is buy less meat.

It takes 2,500 gallons of water to produce just one pound of beef. Compare that to only 100 gallons for one pound of wheat. Those maligned almonds take about 23 gallons of water per ounce. Sounds like a lot, but it's nothing compared to how much water animal products require. Vegetables consume a little over 11,000 gallons of water per ton, while butter, beef, and pork consume 122,800, 145,000, and 121,000 gallons per ton, respectively. Cows lap up 23 gallons of water every single day, while humans consume less than a single gallon. A kilogram of animal protein requires 100 times more water than a kilogram of grain protein. Meanwhile, it takes 132 gallons of water just to slaughter one cow.

Guess which plant sucks up most of California's water supply? Alfalfa. Scratching your head? I mean, who the hell eats alfalfa that much? Hint: not us. Alfalfa takes up more than a million acres of land in California, and it's harvested almost exclusively to feed cows in factory farms. Each cow eats between 25 and 50 pounds of grains/alfalfa a day. In the United States alone we slaughter nearly ninety thousand cows every single day. And if you think grass-fed cow meat is better for your health (it's not), know that it's worse for the environment. Grass-fed cows live eight months longer on average than grain-fed cows—that's eight more months of water, alfalfa, and grains. So if you're concerned how much water your almonds are soaking up, take a closer look at that steak.

But the environmental impacts associated with livestock don't end with water. In fact, the greatest problem might have less to do with the food that goes into the cow than the gas leaving her—methane, that is. Between all the farts from the billions of farm animals reared for slaughter and all the infrastructure associated with moving the world's 275 million tons of meat, the livestock sector generates more greenhouse gases than all CO_2-emitting vehicles combined. Buying a hybrid car is a great choice, but to help combat climate change, the most important step you can take is to eat strong food with roots—roots that can plant a foundation for stopping and even reversing climate change.

Plants are not just health-strong, but also earth-strong.

EAT STRONG FOOD TO STOP AND REVERSE CHRONIC ILLNESS

Heart Disease

Now that you know plants are strong, what is the number one reason to love our strong plants? Because plants are the only way to cure our number one cause of death: heart disease.

That's right—the single biggest reason most Americans are going to die can be eliminated just by eating the right foods. Back when I was a firefighter in Austin, we had to make sure our equipment was in perfect working order. The first thing we would do at our noon shift change was a complete check of all the equipment on the fire engine, from the axes and Halligan tools we carry on the front bumper to the ventilation fans and the medical equipment we carry in the back compartment. We had to make sure everything was in perfect working condition. A ruptured fire hose could mean the difference between saving a house and watching it burn to the ground. If a hose was leaking, we'd never let someone stick his or her finger into the hole or throw some duct tape on it. We'd fix the leak properly and take better care of our hoses so it would never happen again.

The same is true for heart disease. If you've got a ticker at risk of conking out for good, you can throw some duct tape on it with statins and hope for the best. Or you can actually fix the problem by cutting out what caused the problem in the first place: meat, eggs, dairy, fish, processed oils, and processed foods.

This isn't groundbreaking news. We've known for decades how to cure heart disease. In fact, one of the earliest persons to figure it out wasn't even a doctor. He was an engineer named Nathan Pritikin. More than half a century ago he was diagnosed with heart disease at the ripe old age of forty-one. His doctors weren't much more helpful than they are today. Avoid strenuous activity, take the elevator, nap often. Be sure to get your affairs in order. Gee, thanks, Doc.

Pritikin had other ideas. He studied the plant-based eating habits of rural Africans and how they had far fewer instances of heart disease. Pritikin figured that if he stopped eating the junk that made his heart sick, he could make it healthy again. It doesn't take an engineer to put two and two together. (Well, maybe in this case it did.) Pritikin completely changed his diet, and within two years his total cholesterol number dropped from more than 300 to 120. His so-called terminal heart disease vanished. He started to run again, which he hadn't done for years on doctor's orders. He ended up living a normal life.

Some of the more recent scientific proof comes from my father in a follow-up to his 1985 study at the Cleveland Clinic. My dad tracked 198 people who followed similar plant-based eating plans for four years. A staggering 89.3 percent of them stuck to their diets, and in that group only one person suffered another cardiac event (a small stroke). However, among those who returned to their old eating habits, two-thirds of them had another stroke, heart attack, or died. The results were published in the *Journal of Family Practice* in July 2014: "Though current medical and surgical treatments manage coronary artery disease, they do little to prevent or stop it. Nutritional intervention, as shown in our study and others, has halted and even reversed Coronary Artery Disease."

Heart disease is a choice. In other words, it's self-inflicted. This may be hard to swallow, but it's true. These days, though, you'd never know that heart disease was a choice. Let's say you visit your cardiologist, who confirms that you've got a 95 percent blockage in one of the major arteries going to your heart. The first thing he will do is scare you. "We'll need to perform a bypass surgery immediately," he might say, "or else you'll have a heart attack." You'll spend the night in the hospital, and you'll be wheeled into the OR the next morning.

What your doctor didn't tell you is that your 95 percent blockage is actually stable. It's not ideal, and it's not good for your heart in the long term, but it's not likely to cause a heart attack tomorrow. Your amazing body has the capacity to build collateral vessels around the blockage. A surgeon does essentially the same thing by stealing a vein from your leg and grafting it around your blockage to improve blood flow to the heart.

What your surgeon won't tell you, however, is that your vein graft will shut down within eighteen months, and she'll have to perform another procedure. Your doctors also won't tell you that since you have a major blockage in one place, you probably have blockages in dozens of other places in your body. My father has counseled patients who've had up to forty-seven stents put in their arteries. Forty-seven!

A few people have said to me that Rip's diet seemed pretty extreme. I answered with a quote from Rip's dad, Dr. Caldwell Esselstyn: "Having veins taken from your legs and having your chest cracked open for heart surgery is pretty extreme!"

—Alanna Verlei, age 63, retired RN

Of course, no amount of drugs or patch-up plumbing jobs, such as bypass operations, stents, or angioplasties, can do anything to address the underlying cause of heart disease. You fix one blockage, and three more will pop up next month. No degree of surgical whack-a-mole can keep up with heart disease.

What if there were a second option? One without all the pills and surgeries and expensive gadgets that need to be replaced all the time. One that has a nearly 100 percent success rate at stopping and reversing heart disease. It's called changing what you eat. Focusing on strong food will give you the keys to a new health kingdom.

Sounds crazy, but just look around the world. In the famous China Study, for example, researchers led by Dr. T. Colin Campbell followed the mortality rates and eating habits of hundreds of thousands of rural Chinese who ate a primarily plant-based diet. In one province with more than a half million people, not a single death was blamed on heart disease over a period of three years. Meanwhile, in the state of Mississippi alone, heart disease kills more than eight thousand people per year.

But hey, we live in America! We spend more money on medical care than anyone else on the planet. A whopping $3.8 trillion per year! Surely some of that cash must be going to something good. We've got all these patented drugs to keep us alive. Why eat healthy when you can just order a Double Quarter Pounder, a shake, and a side of Lipitor? Because we should know better. Modern medicine is a powerful and appealing distraction that has smart, intelligent people like you falling for it hook, line, and sinker. These pills and procedures are like a seductive mistress pulling people in the wrong direction, toward trouble. If you stay true to your food, heart disease doesn't stand a chance of invading your arteries. That's something I know you can live with!

The CDC (Centers for Disease Control and Prevention) recently noted, "More Americans than ever are taking cholesterol-lowering medications." More than a quarter of adults over forty are taking statins, which helps explain the alarming fact that nearly 70 percent of all Americans are on at least one prescription drug. Overall, doctors are peddling 4 billion prescription drugs every year—the equivalent of thirteen drugs each for every man, woman, and child. The statin Lipitor is the best-selling drug of all time, with more than $140 billion in total sales.

So you arrive for a checkup, your doctor says you've got high cholesterol, and what does she give you? Not some delicious plant-strong recipes to naturally bring down your cholesterol, I can promise you that. She gives you a Lipitor pamphlet.

Your doctor won't tell you that statins have some side effects. For instance, she might order a blood test. Why? Because statins can cause liver toxicity as well as, for some people, severe muscle pain. Moreover, even if your blood work looks normal, biopsies have shown that statins can still be wreaking havoc on your muscles. This is bad news for athletes, and especially bad news for seniors who are at risk of falls. Meanwhile, the Food and Drug Administration recently mandated that labels on statins warn about the very real possibility of memory loss, while a 2013 study among thousands of breast cancer patients in the Seattle–Puget Sound region found that long-term statin use could double a woman's risk of aggressive breast cancer.

These side effects might be tolerable if the drugs really worked, but studies have found that even among high-risk patients, the chance of benefiting from the most common blood pressure, cholesterol, and blood-thinning drugs is less than 5 percent. And statins—the world's most popular drug—may offer only a 3 percent reduction in heart attack risk over six years. After all that money and all those pills and side effects, a measly 3 percent!

It's up to you. Pop a pill, and maybe you'll see a 3 percent chance of getting healthier—that is, if you don't damage your liver, your muscles, and your brain in the process. Pop some plants, and you'll have an almost 100 percent chance of getting healthier. Oh, and did I mention that you'll be actively making your liver, muscles, and brain stronger?

Now you know that a plant-based diet can reverse heart disease, but I'll do you even one better.

You can prevent heart disease before you have to reverse it!

Heart disease, also known as atherosclerosis, is caused by the buildup of fatty deposits called plaque along the walls of your arteries. These deposits increase along with the amount of food you eat that is rich in fat and animal protein.

Now, this doesn't happen all at once. It takes place over decades. Plaque slowly bulges into your arteries, narrowing the space for blood to flow. If a chunk of plaque breaks off and a clot forms, a heart attack can occur. Less severe symptoms include angina, which produces severe chest pains that can radiate to the shoulders, arms, and neck.

However, for some people, the first symptom of heart disease is their final symptom. This is called sudden cardiac death, and it represents about half of all heart disease deaths in the United States. The data tells us that roughly 92 percent of heart attacks are caused by a juvenile plaque that ruptures (like a pimple), followed by the formation of a blood clot. Sudden cardiac death, however, is not actually a heart attack. Instead, the plaque in your arteries kills you over decades by gradually restricting blood flow and damaging the delicate signaling system that tells your heart chambers precisely when to relax and when to pump blood. Suddenly, and without warning, your heart can experience abnormal rhythms called arrhythmias, preventing the flow of blood and killing you.

You get only one heart, though. This means you can't wait until you start feeling symptoms of heart disease to start treating it. With sudden cardiac death, one minute you're feeling 100 percent fine. The next minute, you're dead. That's because your heart disease didn't start a second ago. It probably started during childhood. Autopsies of accidental death victims have discovered that arterial fatty streaks, which are believed to be the precursor to atherosclerosis, are present in almost all American children by age ten! By your thirties, these streaks are turning into sticky, waxy, disgusting plaque. And then...it's only a matter of time.

However, by cutting out all animal products—ideally starting in childhood—you can reverse plaque buildup before it's too late. The body is a miraculous thing, but it can work its magic only if you feed it something equally magical: plants.

PQ Quiz

What's your PQ (plant-quotient) score? Try your hand at these true-or-false questions. You will discover all of the answers after reading part 1, but if you really need to know all the answers now, see page 281.

1. You cannot get enough protein from a plant-based diet because plants do not supply all the essential amino acids.
2. Avocados, extra-virgin olive oil, and coconut oil are all examples of healthy fats.
3. Animal-based foods do not contain any dietary fiber.
4. Plant-based foods do not contain any dietary cholesterol.

5. Dairy products like milk and cheese are the only reliable source of calcium in your diet.
6. Drinking fruit smoothies is just as good as eating whole fruits.
7. One serving of peanut butter is more calorie-dense than a large plate of green salad with no-oil dressing.
8. Apples, broccoli, coconut oil, and organic blue corn chips are all examples of whole plant-based foods.
9. The main reason food can be addictive is because of the high content of salt, sugar, and fat.
10. It is possible to eat a lot of food and still lose weight.
11. Proper diet is more important for overall health than regular exercise.
12. Protein is the most important fuel source for your body.
13. Carbohydrates have the most calories per gram.

Other Killer Diseases

If you think that some fatal disease has you in its crosshairs, I want you to stop this way of thinking immediately.

According to Dr. Michael Greger, director of public health and animal agriculture at the Humane Society of the United States and author (with Gene Stone) of the best-selling book *How Not to Die*, it isn't just our number one killer disease that a plant-based diet can reverse and prevent. A plant-based diet can help you conquer all fifteen leading causes of death in America.

For instance, cancer. More than any other disease, people think of cancer as inevitable—especially if it runs in your family. Your grandma Ruth got it in her seventies, so you're getting it, too. But while genetics can play a role, the truth is, just as with heart disease, you can control your own fate by controlling what you put in your mouth.

Animal products cause cancer by fueling armies of free radicals in your body. Free radicals are like the orcs from *The Lord of the Rings*: they're evil, ugly, and multiply at breakneck speed. What makes these devils so vile and dishonorable is that they feast on something you can't do without—oxygen. Supercharged by electrons that occasionally leak out of your cells, a chance oxygen molecule essentially beefs up on steroids and becomes a free radical. They might sound like a bad '70s rock band, but free radicals aren't so groovy. They're so pumped up with energy that they stampede out of control throughout your cells, smashing and scrambling your DNA and causing cancerous mutations.

Anyone who's ever owned a car fears rust. Like free radicals, rust is caused by exposure to oxygen. That's why the dealer is always trying to sell you the expensive undercoating, so your new rig doesn't rust out from under you. Dad's 1975 Trans Am might look great on the outside, but take a peek underneath and you know the scrap heap is calling.

Free radicals work in a similar way. Animal products laden with saturated fat and trans fat cause inflammation in your body, which unleashes a torrent of free radicals that rot you from within, aging you prematurely and causing cancerous mutations. So that meathead you see in the gym benching 400 pounds and eating three steaks a day might look strong on the outside, but if you look under the hood, everything's rotting away like Dad's Trans Am.

Instead, you need foods that keep you strong on the outside and the inside. You need to eat foods that contain lots of free radical–destroying molecules called antioxidants, which march through your bloodstream and neutralize these ne'er-do-wells before they can damage your DNA.

Think of them as your body's own personal undercoating to keep out the rust. You make some antioxidants naturally, but you need to consume lots of antioxidant-rich food to account for all the free radicals that are produced just by breathing in air. It's a no-brainer which foods are the best—plants average sixty-four times more antioxidants than animal foods.

The evidence is overwhelming. An *International Journal of Cancer* study of nearly a half million people found that the chance of developing pancreatic cancer, which kills 94 percent of people within five years of diagnosis, increases by 72 percent for every 50 grams (or 3 tablespoons) of chicken consumed daily. That's along with at least a 56 percent increased risk of blood cancers including lymphoma and leukemia.

A 2007 study published in the journal *Epidemiology* found that women who consume the most barbecued, grilled, or smoked meat have 47 percent increased odds of developing breast cancer compared to women who eat the least. Among the same group of women, those who ate lots of meat and the least amount of fruits and veggies had 74 percent greater odds of developing breast cancer.

A 2015 meta-analysis (a compilation of many similar studies) published in the *American Journal of Clinical Nutrition* found that the intake of dairy products was directly linked to an increased risk of prostate cancer. Meanwhile, a group of Harvard University researchers studying a thousand men with early-stage prostate cancer found that eating an egg or less a day was associated with twice the risk of cancer progressing to more dangerous stages. Overall, men who consume about an egg every three days may have an 81 percent increased risk of deadly prostate cancer compared to men who don't eat eggs.

It's not genetic. It's diet. Since World War II there's been a nearly twenty-five-fold increase in prostate cancer among men living in Japan. You know what else has gone up? Egg consumption by sevenfold, meat consumption by ninefold, and dairy consumption by twentyfold. You see the same phenomenon with Alzheimer's disease. The rates of this horrendous disease that destroys your brain one memory at a time are four times lower among Africans in Nigeria compared to African Americans living in Indianapolis. Same genetics, different diet. And how about India? The country that eats more grains than any other country has the world's lowest rate of Alzheimer's. Try that one on for size, *grain bashers*!

Now, how about plants? I mentioned earlier that fiber consumption is associated with decreased breast cancer risk. In fact, a *Journal of the National Cancer Institute* review found that for every 20 grams of fiber consumed per day, the risk of breast cancer is reduced by 15 percent— results that have been confirmed in more than a dozen separate studies. (For comparison, the average American consumes a scant 15 grams of fiber daily.) In another study funded by the National Cancer Institute, just 2 teaspoons of ground flaxseeds a day was found to reduce on average the amount of precancerous changes in the breasts of women at high risk of breast cancer—and among breast cancer survivors, those who eat the most flaxseeds appear to live much longer.

A decade ago Dr. Dean Ornish, president and founder of the nonprofit Preventive Medicine Research Institute, decided to shift his focus from his pioneering work on heart disease to cancer. He enlisted 93 men with early-stage "watch-and-wait" prostate cancer and divided them into two groups. The first followed the advice of their current doctors and continued eating the standard American diet, and the second was put on a plant-based diet with lots of fruits, veggies, whole grains, beans, and soy. Guess which group fared better? The first group's PSA levels—an indicator of prostate cancer growth—jumped by 6 percent. But the plant-strong group's PSA levels *dropped* by 4 percent, meaning their tumors began to shrink.

In other words, Dr. Ornish demonstrated that plants can even reverse cancer among people who have it. And that's without blasting your body to smithereens with chemo and undergoing horrendous invasive surgeries.

The largest-ever study of diet and health was conducted by the National Institutes of Health and the American Association of Retired Persons. The NIH-AARP study followed more than 100,000 people for decades. What did this enormous study conclude? "Red and processed meat intakes were associated with modest increases in total mortality, cancer mortality, and cardiovascular disease mortality." *Bam!* Done. You eat more meat, you're more likely to die prematurely. Here is what Dr. Kim Williams, president of the American College of Cardiology, remarked when asked why he doesn't eat meat: "Meat kills you. Processed meat kills you faster. I don't mind dying. I just don't want it to be my fault."

And we're not talking just heart disease and cancer. The bigger the study, the bigger the results. The Harvard Nurses' Health Study followed 16,000 women starting in 1980 and found that those who ate at least one serving of blueberries and two servings of strawberries each week were less likely to experience cognitive decline. A study of 89,000 Californians published in the *American Journal of Clinical Nutrition* found that people who cut out meat, fish, and dairy reduce their risk of type 2 diabetes by 78 percent and their risk of high blood pressure by 75 percent. These two conditions alone kill more than 141,000 Americans each year. The Iowa Women's Health Study, which followed 35,000 women for several decades, concluded that eating green vegetables protects against non-Hodgkin's lymphoma, a very serious blood cancer. Two studies from Harvard and Columbia Universities following a combined 50,000 people found that eating cured meat increases your risk of chronic obstructive pulmonary disease, which affects more than 24 million Americans and kills 134,000 every year.

Before I went to the Engine 2 Diet I would only eat meat at meals. I would very rarely eat vegetables. I have lost over 50 pounds and I am still seeing my weight drop down. I now have more energy and feel great. I always had to keep a bottle of antacids by the bed. Since the change I have not even had any problems with acid reflux. Even though my doctor had diagnosed me with it and had said that I needed to remove anything tomato-based, I now eat meals that have plenty of tomatoes in them and have zero issues.
—Mihail T. Nakoff, age 37, store systems integrator

Preventing chronic disease is great, of course, but what if you've already got one? Plants can still help. We've already seen the miracles they perform against heart disease, but did you know that the spice turmeric is able to reverse precancerous changes in colon cancer, and that lab studies have shown the spice's active ingredient, curcumin, to be effective against lung cancer cells? Did you know that a randomized clinical trial revealed that eating lots of strawberries might be able to reverse the development of esophageal cancer in 80 percent of patients? A 2012 pilot study published in the *Open Journal of Preventive Medicine* found that seven months on a whole-food, plant-based diet could reverse type 2 diabetes entirely—and other studies have found that you can also reverse the painful nerve damage associated with diabetes. In the 1940s, Dr. Walter Kempner, with his famous rice-and-fruit diet, was able to bring patients' blood pressures of near 240/150 down to 105/80.

Trying to prevent a stroke? Eat more strong food. Researchers from Stockholm, Sweden, following 30,000 women determined in 2012 that those who consumed the most antioxidants had the lowest odds of suffering from a stroke. Remember, plant foods average sixty-four times more antioxidants than animal foods.

Hate having to take so many sick days? Broccoli and kale have been found to boost immune system function, and berries can dramatically boost your levels of natural killer cells. They have a badass name for a reason: Natural killer cells are the body's first line of defense against cancerous and virus-infected cells. The more you have, the healthier you stay.

Worried about your liver? Nonalcoholic fatty liver disease (NAFLD) affects some 70 million Americans and can lead to hepatitis, cirrhosis, and eventual liver failure. Want to avoid it? People who eat the meat equivalent of 14 chicken nuggets per day have up to triple the rates of liver disease compared to people who eat fewer than 7 nuggets. Better yet, cut out the KFC altogether—chicken is the number one source of salmonella poisoning and a top source of arachidonic acid, which contributes to severe depression.

What if you just want to lose some weight? That's one of my favorite scenarios, and we'll talk a lot more about it later in the book. With healthy whole foods, you can eat as much as you want and you'll lose that gut! As demonstrated by a 2012 study in the *British Journal of Nutrition*, simply adding beans and other legumes to your diet can promote weight loss just as effectively as cutting 500 calories from your daily diet. Meanwhile, most fruits and vegetables contain between 80 and 90 percent water, which, along with the fiber content, helps you feel full faster (see chapter 3). For example, to equal the amount of calories found in 2 tablespoons of Cheddar cheese (25 grams), you'd have to eat either 30 strawberries, 8 whole tomatoes, or more than a full head of steamed broccoli. Eat more food; lose more weight!

I could go on and on about the amazing, healthy goodness of strong food. I could talk about hundreds of other studies that prove the point. I could talk about all the anecdotal evidence from my own pilot studies, as well as evidence from all the work my dad has done, that proves the point as well. But the bottom line is irrefutable and the scientific evidence is overwhelming: Eating animal products makes you die sooner and die sicker. Eating strong plant foods makes you live longer and live better.

2

Why We Love Whole Foods

Starting your whole-food, plant-strong journey is exhilarating, exciting, and delicious, but almost nobody gets it right from the get-go. This is certainly not your fault. We've all been fed such an overwhelming amount of conflicting messages and ideas about what it means to eat healthy that the vast majority of Americans are confused. In fact, a recent poll asked people which they found easier: doing their taxes or eating a healthy diet. The majority said taxes were easier.

After writing *The Engine 2 Diet*, I asked people to e-mail me at info@engine2.com with questions. I also encouraged people to send me their food logs if they weren't losing weight or getting the results they had hoped for. It was quickly apparent that people didn't understand the difference between eating a junky plant-based diet and eating a *whole-food*, plant-based diet. The good news is that everything about eating whole foods is easy, sensible, and delicious. In this chapter I'm going to underscore the major differences between eating lousy processed plant food and eating healthy, whole, superstrong plant food!

When I receive e-mails like the one below, I realize how easy it is to go astray.

I've been plant-strong since February—but not seeing any results. I don't really like vegetables, and I've been eating a lot of plant-strong processed food like Amy's Burritos, pizzas, Tofurky sandwiches, soy ice-cream, PB&J and pop. I'm hoping I can see some results soon and I want to learn what to eat instead of the frozen meals. Thx.

Pop quiz: name one whole-plant food in that list above. Having trouble? Good. There is no Tofurky plant out there in nature, and Amy's Burritos don't grow naturally in Amy's garden. And I don't even know where to begin when it comes to soy ice cream. The truth is, just because you're not eating animal products doesn't mean you're eating healthy food.

So what does whole food mean, anyway? As Dr. T. Colin Campbell, renowned biochemist and author of the best-selling book *The China Study*, says in *Whole: Rethinking the Science of Nutrition*, "The ideal human diet looks like this: Consume plant-based foods in forms as close to their natural state as possible...Eat a variety of vegetables, fruits, raw nuts and seeds, beans and legumes, and whole grains."

In other words: whole foods are foods in their natural plant form.

Let's take another look at some of those foods mentioned in the e-mail above. Instead of eating Tofurky, why not just eat some tofu, tempeh, or edamame? They're all made directly from whole soybeans, and each has its own unique flavor profile, look, and personality! I'm not even going to ask what was on the pizza besides the starchy, processed white flour and cheese, all soaking in treacherous oils. Meanwhile, that peanut butter and jelly sandwich may well be the most calorie-dense snack you can eat other than sipping pure oil.

Just because a food is technically plant-based does not make it plant-*strong*. Darth Vader is technically Anakin Skywalker, but he's been so deformed by the dark side that he bears no resemblance to his former self. Processed foods are the Darth Vader of plants. French fries are technically potatoes, but these poor potatoes have been abused and distorted and corrupted—that is, "processed"—into French fries. We take the almighty potato, which in 2008 was deemed vegetable of the year by the World Health Organization, and torture the poor thing until it's lost almost all of its nutritional integrity. With a little help from the deep fryer, this lean and strong vegetable, containing only 2 percent fat, turns into a weak food that's now 51 percent fat, showered in salt, and ultimately dipped into another corrupted, processed, and adulterated vegetable: ketchup, which is typically laden with high-fructose corn syrup or cane sugar.

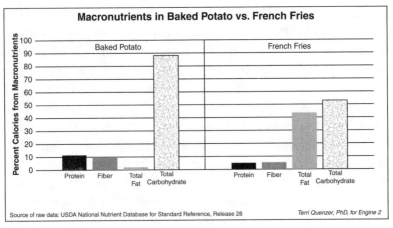

As a famous rock star once said, "I'd rather be baked than fried!"

On the other hand, a whole baked potato, with its nutritious skin intact, has more vitamin C than an orange, more potassium than a banana, and as much fiber as a bowl of oatmeal.

Take another turn through the grocery store and you'll see an entire aisle of so-called healthy plant-based products. For example, many people think that Daiya cheese, a popular cheese alternative, must be healthy because it's nondairy. But Daiya is actually 70 percent fat, and the second ingredient staring up at you without a shred of guilt is canola oil. Earth Balance spread is making the rounds as healthier than butter, but it has the same number of calories per tablespoon (100) as butter, and the first ingredient is an expeller-pressed natural oil blend (soybean, palm, canola, olive). The product is 100 percent fat. Why is this healthy?

Here's what I mean by eating whole foods. Instead of sodium- and sugar-rich tomato juice, just eat a whole tomato, perhaps with a drizzle of balsamic vinegar and a dash of pepper. Instead of that processed sugar bomb they call Raisin Bran, just have some oatmeal, quinoa, or rice like the recipes on pages 197–204. Instead of eating vegetable chips that are chirping with added sugar, salt, and oils, go out and gorge on some whole vegetables.

These days only about 6 percent of Americans' calories come from whole-plant foods such as broccoli, brown rice, wheat berries, bananas, oranges, apples, beans, and potatoes. Over the next seven days I want you to swing that plant-strong pendulum around so instead of a paltry 6 percent, you're moving it to DEFCON 1 and calories that are a full 100 percent plant-based. I want you to be adventurous with meals, including baked potato and sweet potato bowls with brown rice, bell peppers, scallions, steamed kale, and a clean red sauce like the Red Pepper Hummus on page 261. In fact, we like sweet potatoes anytime of the day, as the foundation in a breakfast bowl (see pages 194–204), with the Chopped and Cubed Salad (page 211), or in the Sweet Potato Bowl (page 237). With the Engine 2 Rescue Diet, the food you eat is in its whole form, not isolated bits and scraps that have zero nutritional value.

In other words, just because a food is plant-based doesn't mean it's healthy. There are plenty of plant-based junk foods out there. For example, what about the "certified vegan" Dr. Praeger's Thai Veggie Burgers? Mother Nature certainly didn't certify this food: One patty's got nearly 200 mg of sodium, 8 grams of fat, and a long ingredients list that includes canola oil. Despite all that processing, it is health*ier* than a real hamburger, but that doesn't mean it's strong-food healthy.

So be vigilant. Don't be fooled by frozen vegan entrées that have more sodium than the Red Sea; vegan buttery spreads that have more fat than Fat Albert; vegan chips and crackers that have more oil than the Arabian Peninsula; vegan cookies and cakes that have more sugar than a Krispy Kreme factory; and vegan hot dogs, hamburgers, and other pseudomeats that have more isolated soy proteins than a tub of muscle milk.

No matter what the label says, highly processed foods aren't your friend, even if they're technically plant-based. They are your foe, and I want you to steer clear of them over the next seven days. In the best-case scenario, these empty foods are missing vitamins, minerals, fiber, and other nutrients. In the worst case, they actively promote the development of chronic disease and fuel existing chronic conditions and disease. Meanwhile, we drink almost 25 percent of our calories (you will be reading more about this in chapter 3); we put processed and extracted oils in and on everything just like the big food manufacturers do, which accounts for another 20 to 25 percent of our calories; and we consume 40 teaspoons of added sweeteners daily, which is another 25 percent of our calories.

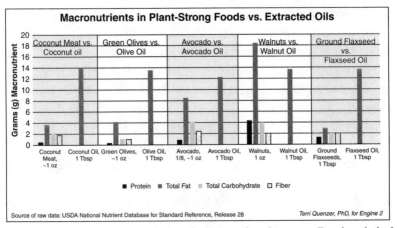

This is why all oils are black holes of nutritional nothingness. Eat the whole food for maximum nutritional oomph!

In his book *The Campbell Plan*, T. Colin Campbell's son, Dr. Tom Campbell, refers to processed and refined plant foods as "plant fragments." When you take a closer look at how America eats, you realize that the majority of our calories are coming from three ingredients: white flour, white sugar, and oil. As dietician Jeff Novick likes to say, when you bake all three of these together, you get one big donut. And that's essentially where the vast majority of America's calories are coming from—processed and refined flour, sugar, and oils. America lives on one big donut, and our collective health reflects just that!

Instead, bring on the whole foods and let's ditch the processed plant fragments. Be strong and eat whole, strong-plant foods!

When Vegan Isn't Healthy

Maybe the only thing I hate as much as animal products pretending to be healthy are vegan products pretending to be healthy. Remember, just because it's technically plant-based doesn't mean it's plant-strong. Take Pop-Tarts, for example. Not exactly anyone's idea of a balanced, nutritious breakfast, but they're technically vegan. One frosted strawberry tart has 16 grams of sugar, 170 mg of sodium, and less than 1 gram of fiber while having more ingredients than rocket fuel, some with names like "red 40" and "modified wheat starch." What the heck does *modified* actually mean?

The first ingredient is enriched flour, which shouldn't come as a big surprise. Most people who buy Pop-Tarts aren't looking for a 100 percent whole-grain product. However, the second, third, fourth, and sixth ingredients are four different kinds of added sugar: corn syrup, high-fructose corn syrup, dextrose, and sugar. How many added teaspoons of sugar are in one Pop-Tart? Let's do the math. The nutrition facts panel states that there are 16 grams of sugar in one Pop-Tart. Since there are 4 grams of sugar per teaspoon, that means one Pop-Tart contains a whopping 4 teaspoons of sugar. The fifth ingredient is a combination of soybean oil and palm oil. Can we all say "inflammatory unhealthy fats" at once?

How about kale chips? You'd think they'd have to be healthy, right? Guess again. A single 1-ounce serving of store-bought kale chips may contain 160 calories, 10 grams of fat, and 150 mg of sodium. Meanwhile, 1 ounce of unprocessed raw kale has 14 calories, 0.2 gram of fat, and 12 mg of sodium. Oops again.

The bottom line: junk food is junk food, plant-based or not.

During the Rescue Week we are focused on eating 100 percent plant-based foods that are as minimally processed as possible....This means as close to grown as possible. This is why I want to make it super clear: No oil! None! Unless the oil occurs naturally in strong whole foods, don't go near it!

Let's keep this one simple, because I'm tired of repeating it: *all processed oil is unnecessary and unhealthy!*

Wait a minute. What about olive oil? Olive oil comes from olives. Olives are plants. Therefore, olive oil is good for you, right?

Wrong!

Not a chance!

Ain't gonna fly!

Now, I don't want all the folks who live and die by their extra-virgin olive oil to curse me and throw this book out the window. Let's take a deep breath and take a closer look at olive oil so we can understand why it isn't the miracle health product you've been led to believe.

When you squeeze the oil out of olives to make olive oil, you end up with a concentrated source of calories that is 100 percent fat and devoid of almost all vitamins and minerals. Just a single tablespoon of olive oil contains about 120 empty calories. Did you know that it takes more than 1,300 olives to produce a single 32-ounce bottle of olive oil? Meanwhile, 1 innocent little tablespoon of olive oil is the fat equivalent of about 45 olives (and a black hole of nutritional nothingness).

Some olive-oil lovers out there like to say, "Hey, wait a minute, Rip. Olive oil has vitamins E and K. How can you say olive oil is entirely empty calories?" Okay, you got me. You're right. It's true, olive oil does have trace amounts of those vitamins…but you'd have to guzzle 10 tablespoons of it to meet your daily requirement for both. You'd also have to guzzle *half a pound of olive oil*—about 2,000 calories' worth—in order to reach your daily recommended intake of omega-3 fatty acids. I can't think of a better way to stop your heart than by quaffing down a half pound of oil!

What about Coconut Oil?

Boy, do I get this one a lot. For some reason, these days coconut oil is being touted as a wonder cure for everything from Alzheimer's to heart disease to obesity, due to its alleged antimicrobial abilities.

Let me repeat: *All oil is junk.* Like all oils, coconut oil is stripped of nearly all nutrients. Instead of the healthy fiber you'd receive from eating the meat of a coconut, you get globs of saturated fat, which acts the exact same way as the inflammation-promoting saturated fat in olive oil and all animal products.

In an interview with the *New York Times*, Dr. Alice H. Lichtenstein, a professor of nutrition science and policy at Tufts University and vice-chair of the federal government's dietary guidelines advisory committee, said that despite "a lot of hype about [coconut oil] there's virtually no data to support the hype."

Worst of all, the long-chain saturated fatty acids in coconut oil promote bad cholesterol, evidenced by a randomized study published in the *American Journal of Clinical Nutrition* that found that regularly ingesting coconut oil can significantly raise your LDL ("bad") cholesterol levels. This makes sense because coconut oil is an artery-busting 92 percent saturated fat—more than any other food on the planet! Gram for gram, that's more saturated fat than butter, lard, or beef fat. In another study, published in the journal *Lipids*, subjects placed on a weight-loss diet were also given coconut oil. Despite losing weight, their LDL cholesterol levels actually increased—when you lose weight naturally, the opposite is supposed to happen.

It's not good for your heart and it's not good for your food. Coconut oil is just another snake oil, as far as I'm concerned. I don't care if your coconuts or olives or corn or peanuts were planted in the Garden of Eden and watered with Eve's tears—no matter where it came from, *all oil is junk*!

But the calories that olive oil contains are not just empty calories—they're downright *dangerous* calories. As I've mentioned many times to many people, noted physiologist Ray Peat has written, "All oils, even if they're organic, cold-pressed, unprocessed, bottled in glass, and stored away from heat and light, are damaging. These oils have no shelf life at all...and when they're warmed to body temperature, they disintegrate even faster. Once ingested, they bind with cells and interfere with every chemical reaction in the body. The results are hormone imbalances, inflammation, and all kinds of illness."

And don't believe those "heart-healthy" labels you see on olive oil containers. While olive oil might technically be better than, say, corn oil or canola oil, that doesn't make it healthy. That's like Philip Morris saying their cigarettes are healthy because they have filters. In fact, olive oil is the opposite of heart-healthy. A study published in the journal *Clinical Cardiology* found that olive oil significantly hindered the ability of people's arteries to dilate. In other words, oil restricts blood flow to and from the heart.

Similar studies have shown that blood flow decreases drastically for many hours after a fatty meal. Is it any wonder that so many of us "crash" after a heavy meal? It's also no wonder that, as Brigham and Women's Hospital researchers reported after studying more than 2,000 cardiac patients, the risk of heart attack jumps by 400 percent immediately following a heavy, fat-rich meal. And how many of us down a heavy, fat-rich meal for breakfast, lunch, and dinner year after year and decade after decade? Lots!

Think about the water pipes in your house. Normally, water flows freely through the pipes and out your faucets. Now, what happens if you pour oil into the water supply? The thick, viscous oil clogs the pipes, slowing the flow to a crawl. In fact, a notice in our Austin, Texas, utility bill asked us not to pour oil and grease down the sink because of the damage it does to water pipes. Blood vessels are just like water pipes: blood should flow freely and unobstructed, like water. But adding oils to your diet clogs your body's own plumbing, impairing the ability of your vessels to deliver nutrients throughout the body and to supply your cells with oxygen.

Oil consumption leads to inflammation and plaque buildup no matter how healthy you may look and feel. A study published in the *Journal of the American College of Nutrition* revealed that a high-fat diet boosted inflammatory proteins in the blood by 25 percent even though the study subjects lost weight. Conversely, among subjects who lost the same amount of weight on a low-fat, high-carb diet, inflammatory protein levels *dropped* by 43 percent. The resulting inflammation leads to heart disease.

For example, a study by University of Crete researchers found that Crete residents with the highest intake of monounsaturated fats, primarily from olive oil, were far more likely to have heart disease. Another study, this one published in the *Journal of the American Medical Association*, determined that all oils—including saturated, monounsaturated (olive oil), and polyunsaturated (flax oil)—were associated with an increase in the plaque buildup that clogs arteries and leads to heart attacks. To add insult to injury, according to the National Institutes of Health, oil suppresses your immune system, which makes you vulnerable to infections and impairs your body's ability to stop the growth of cancer cells.

Enough is enough. Let's keep this simple. Oil is for car engines, not human bodies. Don't dip in it, drip it, pour it, mix it, drizzle it, cook it, or buy products with it. As my father says, oil is the "gateway to vascular disease. It doesn't matter whether it's olive oil, corn oil, coconut oil, canola oil, or any other kind. Avoid ALL oil."

Cooking without Oil

I get this question all the time: Can you still cook with oil?

Not during your Rescue Week!

In addition to the heart disease–promoting problems with using oil (aka liquid fat), cooking with oil over high heat can alter its chemical composition, which may give rise to toxins called peroxides that cause cancer-causing DNA mutations.

Don't worry, though. You can still be a gourmet cook and never touch oil. Contrary to popular belief, you won't need a spatula to scrape your scorched veggies off the pan. In fact, it's super easy to cook your favorite, mouthwatering, plant-strong dishes without oil.

Baking. You don't need oil to give your veggies that lovely brown crisp. They will brown just fine on their own as long as you reduce the heat slightly, place them on parchment paper, and let them roast for a little while longer.

Sautéing. You don't need oil to get that beautiful golden brown when sautéing veggies, either. They will brown just as nicely without the added disease-causing fat calories. Onions will sauté entirely by themselves and caramelize on their own in a nonstick pan over medium-high heat after 5 to 7 minutes. Additionally, you can add a few dashes of vegetable broth, orange juice, or simply water. Make sure to stir continuously.

Stir-Frying. Stir-frying is the process of cooking food rapidly in a hot wok or skillet, with each ingredient added in rapid-fire succession. If you're not careful, this is one of the easiest ways to turn a seemingly healthy dish into a horrific fat-infused death meal. One teaspoon of oil can quickly turn into a tablespoon, which can quickly turn into a cup. (Just check out any cooking show and see how the chef pours in pints of olive oil when preparing recipes!) Instead, get your wok or skillet nice and hot and then add a few tablespoons of veggie broth. Add in your vegetables and stir continuously. Also try using carrot juice, apple cider, beer, or wine.

Steaming. This might be one of the easiest and simplest ways to cook your veggies. Find a steamer basket and place it at the bottom of a nice big pot or skillet. Add water until it's level with the bottom of the basket. Wait until the water is boiling and then toss your veggies into the basket. Don't overcook, or you risk turning your veggies into a pile of mush. We have a neat trick for you to use when cooking broccoli, on page 265, which I suggest you try several times during the seven days.

We don't need oil to cook anymore! I'm not sick to my stomach after eating. I am always satisfied! Tired of chewing so much, but satisfied!

—Heather Gorski, age 34, teacher

I think my biggest discovery during the Rescue Week is that you can actually cook without oil!

—Judy Watters, age 63, photographer

WHOLE FOODS HAVE STRONG AND MOBILE FIBER

Plants are the Big Daddy when it comes to fiber, which comes in two forms: soluble and insoluble. Soluble fiber dissolves in water and is found in foods such as oats, nuts, beans, barley, flax, carrots, apples, and oranges. Insoluble fiber doesn't dissolve in water. It moves intact through the body and is found in leafy greens, root veggies, and whole-grain foods.

Both forms of fiber are essential, and no matter which kind you choose, plants are fiber kings. Then again, there isn't much competition: There's zero fiber in meat. Zero in dairy products. Zero in eggs.

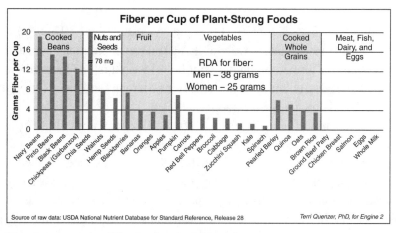

There's a mountain of fiber in plant-based foods!

Why eat fiber? Well, the number one reason is all about number two. Eat plants and discover a world in which constipation is a thing of the past. That's right: Fiber is essential in keeping you unclogged and regular. It's the key to a symbiotic and loving relationship with your intestinal tract.

Fiber is the indigestible stuff of plant food that sticks around with you from mouth to toilet, absorbing water toxins along the way and making your bowel movements easy like Sunday morning. And I don't want to hear any crap about having to go to the bathroom more often. In general, the more often you poop, the healthier you are. If you're squatting on the john fewer than three times per week, you're officially suffering from constipation. Your bowel movements should happen daily, and, ideally, more than once. Consider this a newfound blessing and count each one as such; most people are cursed with a broken-down gastrointestinal tract and are in a world of hurt caused by the wrong, weak, fiberless foods.

> Ah, the glory of a nice body-emptying bowel movement. They are now fuller and have better consistency. Gone are the "rabbit pellets" I had to work at forcing out!
> —Mark Longfellow, age 49, software test analyst

And don't just poop often. Poop big. As one study by University of Cambridge researchers involving twenty-three populations across a dozen countries found, the lighter your bowel weight is, the more likely you are to develop colon cancer. That's right—strong food means strong big wonderful cow-patty-size poops!

The benefits of fiber don't just affect your rear end. High fiber intake has also been shown to control cholesterol, blood sugar, and blood pressure levels, and to reduce the risk of breast cancer, diabetes, heart disease, and obesity. Boosting your fiber intake by 7 grams a day can reduce your risk of stroke by 7 percent—that's just one serving of baked beans. In a recent study, Yale University researchers found that premenopausal women eating more than 6 grams a day of soluble fiber (just a cup of black beans) had 62 percent lower odds of breast cancer when compared with women who ate less than 4 grams.

A Healthy Microbiome!

We are just now beginning to understand the relationship between a healthy microbiome—that is, the microorganisms that live inside us—and what we choose to eat. Mladen Golubic, MD, PhD, and medical director of the Lifestyle 180 program at the Cleveland Clinic's Wellness Institute, has this to say on the health of our guts:

> When we consider making healthy dietary choices, our focus is on potential benefits to life-sustaining functions of our organs, human organs, that is. This diet may be good for my brain, that one for my heart, while the third one may keep my kidney- or liver-associated functions optimal. Until very recently, it did not even cross our minds to include the well-being of a very special "organ" within our gut composed of cells of microorganisms, not our human cells…
>
> An intricate and complex network of a variety of microbes that are adapted to each other and live in our gut affect many physiological functions of humans, from nutrient absorption to fermentation of dietary fiber to help with development and regulation of the immune system and protection from invading disease-causing microorganisms. It is well established that a spectrum of preventable chronic, noncommunicable diseases, such as cardiovascular disease, obesity, certain common types of cancer, autoimmune diseases etc., are associated with gut microbial imbalances, both in the type, number and

biological diversity of microbial species. For example, it is well established that people with low diversity of gut microorganisms have a higher level of body fat and inflammation than those with a rich gut microbial life...

A simple switch from a fully animal-based diet to a fully plant-based diet changes the abundance of certain types of microorganisms leading to decreased inflammation, the underlying driver of multiple chronic diseases... It is clear that increased intake of plant-foods is the best way to avoid starvation of our microbial friends and in turn keep microbial/our own metabolism healthy.

Indeed, studies in the journals *Nature* and *Science* have revealed that the entire human population can essentially be divided into two distinct groups: people whose gut bacteria consist predominantly of *Bacteroides* and people with gut bacteria consisting of *Prevotella*. Interestingly, the type of organisms living in your body isn't related to your body type, gender, or age. Rather, it's dependent on what you eat.

People with guts full of *Bacteroides* are much more likely to consume food components overwhelmingly found in animal foods—such as fat and protein—while people with *Prevotella* guts have food components found in plants—such as fiber and carbohydrates. For example, large-scale studies have found that plant-based African populations are predominantly *Prevotella* while African Americans on the standard American diet are *Bacteroides*. Guess which microbiome is healthier? You guessed it: *Prevotella* prevails! *Bacteroides* guts are associated with a higher risk of colon cancer. An article in the *Journal of Nutrition* points out that African Americans develop colon cancer at fifty times the rate of native Africans.

As I've discussed in my previous books, one of the many disastrous consequences of following the standard American diet is eating minimal to no fiber. On day one of the Seven-Day Rescue, you'll start consuming between 50 and 75 grams of fiber every single day! As one of our pilot study participants said, "I consumed more fruits and vegetables on the first day of this program than I had the previous month!" And when you eat whole, plant-strong food with all of its glorious fiber naturally intact, you'll be forming a whole new relationship with your gastrointestinal tract, your colon, and your rectum. They will thank you for greasing up the skids with plant fiber, and you'll be thanking them for the money you'll be saving at CVS and Walgreens.

Constipation

Sometimes the breathtaking results of switching to a plant-strong diet are best told by Seven-Day Rescue Diet participants in their own words.

I had a woman in the program named Tara Peet, age 36, whose results over the seven days were "effin' fantastic!" She wrote:

> My total cholesterol went from 251 to 190, my LDL cholesterol went from 141 to 103, my triglycerides went from 297 to 128, and I lost 10 pounds. You've got to be kidding me!
>
> Not only do I poop like a champion, I'm pooping all the time and it's the kind of poop where there is barely any wiping involved. Just a nice clean, glorious poop! I have more energy and that is something you need when you have a child. I wasn't sold on this until I saw the results of just seven days.

Here's another letter, by Lori Mills, age 48, outpatient registrar:

> I suffered from severe chronic constipation for over ten years. I have taken prescription stool softeners,

laxatives, antibiotic suppositories for fissures, and Lidocaine gel to numb the pain. Even after a fissurectomy and sphincterotomy I still had all of these issues.

My movements were still dizzyingly painful. Even the muscle flexing involved in passing gas is painful when the rectum is so inflamed and damaged. During about two years of this roughly decade-long period, I was also taking Vicodin and Flexeril three times a day for a work-related back injury.

Then I was introduced to the Engine 2 program. Giving up the meat was not so bad, but I missed dairy. However, within three days of eating plant-strong I had a comfortable bowel movement. Within five days I was having regular, comfortable, and blood-free bowel movements. By the end of twenty-eight days I was hemorrhoid-free.

Whole Grains

I'm sick to my stomach with all this anticarbohydrate propaganda that's been making the rounds lately. Listen up: Carbs are an absolutely essential part of your diet. Without them, you die. No carbs, no energy. What you should be careful of, however, is where you get them from— namely, get them from whole grains, not from processed grains.

Whole grains are an essential part of a healthy diet. Just look at the evidence. Two massive Harvard University studies following nearly 120,000 people for about fifteen years found that those who eat lots of whole grains are much more likely to live longer. That's probably because whole grains can reduce your risk of heart disease, obesity, type 2 diabetes, and stroke, among many other chronic diseases.

Notice I said *whole* grains, not *processed* grains or *refined* grains.

But what are whole grains, exactly? At the grocery store, it's hard to tell which products are healthy and which aren't. Here's a hint: Just because a product's label says "wheat" doesn't mean it's healthy. Subway likes to sell you on its "nine-grain wheat bread," but it's just as refined and sugar-laden as its other breads. Likewise, you'll see all sorts of "multigrain" and "rustic-wheat" bread products at the store that purport to be healthy, but they're just loaves of crap.

Genuine whole grains are unrefined, which means they haven't had their bran (the outer layer of the grain) and germ (the tiny nugget nestled deep inside the grain) removed. You know, the nutritious parts. Imagine gutting the inside of a Rolex. The watch might still look the same on the outside, but the essential parts are no longer there. That's what happens with refined grains. Both the bran and the germ are torn out of the grain, not to mention other essential nutrients like fiber. Why would food manufacturers do such a horrible thing?

Removing the bran and the germ greatly extends the shelf life of the bread, that's why. Grocery stores can pack their shelves with white bread, white rice, pasta, muffins, breakfast cereals, and countless other products. But while food manufacturers are padding their bottom line, the rest of us are left padding our bottoms. That's because refined grains are stripped of satiating fiber, which leads to overeating and weight gain. Try bingeing on oatmeal sometime. Good luck with that, since all that fiber fills you up fast. The opposite happens with processed carbs. Try watching people down breadsticks and pasta Alfredo by the bowl at the Olive Garden. Their bodies are craving what little fiber these impostor grains have, and the result is weight gain. It should be no surprise, therefore, that a meta-analysis in the *European Journal of Epidemiology* found that eating whole grains is associated with a much lower risk of developing type 2 diabetes.

Here's my rule: Don't trust what manufacturers say on their packaging. Anything that screams multigrain, natural-wheat, seven-grain, snap-crackle-and-pop grain—or whatever those marketing geniuses come up with—is probably bunk. Leave it on the shelf. Food companies are getting even sneakier these days by using raisin juice and other food dyes to turn their Frankenstein loaf into a healthy-looking shade of brown. Just because it looks healthy doesn't mean it is healthy!

Here's another simple rule: If the ingredients list is longer than your shopping list, stay far away. For example, here are some of the ingredients from good old all-American Wonder Bread:

High-fructose corn syrup, wheat gluten, salt, soybean oil, yeast, calcium sulphate, vinegar, monoglyceride, dough conditioners (sodium stearoyl lactylate, calcium dioxide), soy flour, diammonium phosphate, dicalcium phosphate, monocalcium phosphate, yeast nutrients (ammonium sulfate), calcium propionate

Now compare that to the ingredients list of oatmeal:

Oats

It has only one ingredient because you're eating the whole food: oats from the oat plant. There's no Wonder Bread flower, a muffin bush, or a vine of Little Debbies.

That said, not all packaged grain products are necessarily bad, but how do you tell the difference? For the answer, let's call in Patrick Skerrett, coauthor of *Eat, Drink, and Be Healthy: The Harvard Medical School Guide to Healthy Eating* and the former executive editor of Harvard Health Publications. Patrick recommends a 1:10 rule: For every 10 grams of carbs per serving in a product, there should be at least 1 gram of fiber. As Patrick writes:

That's about the ratio of fiber to carbohydrate in a genuine whole grain...Divide the grams of carbohydrates by 10. If the [number of] grams of fiber is at least as large as the answer, the food meets the 1:10 standard. I find this a lot easier than reading through an ingredient list, which can be long and baffling (plus there are at least 29 different whole grains that can appear in the ingredients list).

Let's put Patrick's rule into action. One Thomas' English Muffin has 25 grams of carbohydrates and 1 gram of fiber. If you divide the number of carbs (25) by 10, you get 2.5, more than your muffin's 1 gram of fiber. Ezekiel Sprouted Whole Grain English Muffins, on the other hand, have 15 grams of carbs to 3 grams of fiber. If you divide the number of carbs (15) by 10, you get 1.5. Boom, your 3 grams of fiber is bigger. Much better. How about our old pal Wonder Bread? Thirteen grams of carbs to *0* grams of fiber. Yup, zero.

How about rice? Considering that rice alone feeds half the human population, it is one of the most important foods in the world. And this little grain can be extremely healthy, too, but only if you pick the right kind. It comes down to whether you're eating strong brown rice or weak white rice.

Producing brown rice—or strong rice, as I call it—involves removing only the outermost hull of the grain, and nothing more. The germ and the bran remain intact, not to mention the layer of healthy essential fats. By eating strong rice, you are eating all the strong vitamins and minerals that are associated with the whole food, including manganese, selenium, phosphorus, copper, magnesium, and vitamin B_3.

Now let's look at weak—that is, white—rice. You'll agree that it's weak once you see just how deprived this so-called food is. After removing the hull, the rice grain is further milled to remove the bran and nearly all the germ—and just about all the nutrition. Then the rice is "polished" to improve shelf life, a euphemism for stripping the grain of its aleurone layer, which is filled with essential fats. You're left with a white, almost translucent appearance, which makes sense since there's basically nothing left in the rice but starch. Compared to strong brown rice, weak white rice loses 67 percent of vitamin B_3, 80 percent of vitamin B_1, 90 percent of vitamin B_6, 50 percent of manganese, 50 percent of phosphorus, and 60 percent of iron. Weak rice also loses 100 percent of its fiber and nearly all its essential fatty acids.

In 2012, a meta-analysis of seven separate studies following 350,000 people for twenty years was published in the *BMJ* (*British Medical Journal*). It found that people eating higher amounts of white rice had a significantly higher risk of developing type 2 diabetes. In fact, each additional serving of white rice was associated with an 11 percent increased risk of diabetes. You eat weak rice, it makes you weak. End of story.

Harvard University researchers similarly found that a daily serving of white rice was associated with a 17 percent greater risk of developing diabetes, but replacing just one-third of that serving with brown rice could lead to a 16 percent *decrease* in diabetes risk. In addition, due to its high fiber content, brown rice has been shown to decrease the risk of colon cancer as well as many other chronic diseases. Now that's what I call a strong food!

In Part 2 you'll find all sorts of plant-strong recipes centered around whole grains, especially the most muscularly strong food of them all— oatmeal! Not only does oatmeal help protect you against diabetes, obesity, heart disease, cancer, and many other chronic diseases, but it can actively help someone suffering from a chronic disease.

A double-blind, randomized, placebo-controlled trial (the gold standard for clinical trials), published in *Plant Foods for Human Nutrition*, emphatically proved that simply adding oatmeal to your diet can reduce the amount of liver inflammation, not to mention help you lose weight. A follow-up study published in 2014 by the *European Journal of Nutrition* verified these results and further concluded that adding refined grains to your diet instead actively *increases* your chance of liver disease.

Don't Eat Plant Pills

We've talked about all the wonderful health-promoting vitamins, minerals, antioxidants, and phytonutrients that are in plants. But supplement manufacturers think they can harness the awesome power of Mother Nature and jam it all into a little pill. It doesn't work. The tens of thousands of nutrients in plants work synergistically to fight cancer and heart disease and countless other chronic diseases; you can't merely isolate one specific nutrient and expect it to work wonders on its own.

For example, a study published in the *International Journal of Cancer* found that while taking in lots of vitamin C naturally with fruits and veggies can lower your lymphoma risk, taking a vitamin C supplement has no effect at all. Similarly, consuming the B vitamin folate found in whole-plant foods like beans and greens has been shown to lower your risk of depression, while folate supplements have absolutely zero effect on your mood.

In fact, taking isolated, artificially created nutrients in extremely high doses can be detrimental to your health. A meta-analysis published in the *Lancet* found that consuming high individual amounts of vitamin A, vitamin E, and beta-carotene in pill form actually helped "increase overall mortality" among the 170,000 people analyzed.

How about two other popular supplements: fish oil and calcium? Well, science hasn't been kind to them, either. The Diet and Angina Randomized Trial (DART-2), which followed more than 3,000 men, found that participants told "to eat oily fish or take fish oil" actually had a higher risk of cardiac death than those who were not instructed to do so. Moreover, a study published in the *Journal of the National Cancer Institute* determined that men with high amounts of the long-chain omega-3 fat DHA in their blood—which is found in many fish oil supplements—had a higher risk of developing prostate cancer compared to men with low amounts of DHA in their blood.

As far as calcium pills are concerned, a 2011 study in the *BMJ* concluded that these supplements "modestly increase the risk of cardiovascular events," including heart attack and stroke. And here's the real kicker: A 2007 study published in the *American Journal of Clinical Nutrition* reported that "pooled results from randomized controlled trials show no reduction in hip fracture risk with calcium supplementation, and an increased risk is possible." Oh well!

The only supplement plant-based eaters should take is vitamin B_{12}, which is found naturally in soil and made by microorganisms. We used to get it from our water supply and from the dirt clinging to our fresh vegetables just out of the ground, but modern chlorination and packing practices kill off all bacteria. That's no problem, however, because you can easily take a 250 mcg supplement daily (or two 1000 mcg pills twice a week). Alternatively, you can dip into the wealth of B_{12}-fortified grains and nondairy (unsweetened) milks available at the grocery store.

Once you remove all processed foods from your diet, the change in your health will be instant and it will be dramatic. That might be what I love most about plant-based eating. Between 2002 and 2011, nutrition expert Dr. John McDougall put 1,615 patients, most with a history of chronic ailments such as high cholesterol and hypertension, on a crash seven-day program not unlike the Engine 2 Rescue Diet. Dr. McDougall's patients were given whole-plant foods only—no meat, fish, eggs, dairy, or isolated vegetable oils. Instead, the meals were based around healthy carbohydrates including brown rice, oats, barley, quinoa, and potatoes, along with plenty of fruit and beans. There was no portion control or calorie counting. Only whole foods.

In just those seven days, the median weight loss was 3 pounds, and the median decrease in total cholesterol was 22 mg/dl (and a drop of 39 mg/dl among the most unhealthy patients). Patients with the highest initial blood pressure saw their systolic pressure drop by 18 mm/Hg and their diastolic pressure by 11 mm/Hg. Among those on diabetes or blood pressure medication upon entering the program, nearly 90 percent reduced their dosage or discontinued the meds entirely. And if that's what happens after just seven days of eating nothing but whole foods, imagine what will happen over an entire lifetime.

The bottom line: Refined foods will make you weak and sickly. Whole foods will make you strong and healthy. And that's nothing but the *whole truth.*

I'd always thought that heart disease was hereditary and that I'd suffer the fate of my father, who died of a massive heart attack at age fifty-five. When I learned that heart disease was actually preventable through a plant-based diet, changing my eating habits became a no-brainer.

It was a little over three years ago when my annual physical for work (I'm a police officer) revealed that my cholesterol was high. I was urged to start taking statins. *I'm not even forty years old!* I thought. I was certainly not ready to start taking daily medications and endure their unpleasant side effects for the rest of my life. Around the same time, my wife's employer sponsored a wellness initiative that focused on plant-based eating. She shared what she was learning and it really resonated with me. I watched *Forks over Knives* and discovered that heart disease is essentially self-inflicted and *not* hereditary! I immediately felt a sense of relief knowing that I had control of my health and would not be destined to the same fate as my father.

I immediately decided to convert to a plant-based diet (with little to no encouragement from my cardiologist). Food became my medicine! In eight months, my cholesterol dropped from 240 to 141 and I lost more than 30 pounds. I've never looked back!

—Kevin White, age 42, police sergeant

3

Why We Don't Drink Our Food

I bet I know what you're thinking: *Liquid food? Who in the world actually drinks their food?*

The problem is, lots of people do. In fact, Americans drink an alarming amount of their calories—between a quarter to one-half of their entire daily intake. And I'm not just talking about sugary sodas and milk shakes and other weak liquids that we already know are unhealthy. I'm talking about beverages that masquerade as healthy strong food.

Not long ago I received an e-mail from Pamela, a woman in California who was just beginning her plant-strong journey. She wrote:

> I have been 110 percent plant-strong and I have lost NO weight. I am in the gym 8 hours a week!! I am very upset and don't think this is for everyone!!

I asked Pamela for her food journal, and this is what she sent back:

> **Breakfast:** Oatmeal with honey, dried fruit, almond butter, and almond milk.
> **Lunch:** Usually Amy's frozen meals, veggie dogs, Subway veggie sandwich with a little mayo and avocado.
> **Smoothies:** Vega protein powder with essential oils 3X day.
> **Dinner:** I only use extra-virgin olive oil and make stir-fries or frozen meals. I also occasionally eat pork and sometimes fish, but I'm still plant-strong.

Dessert: I haven't found any vegan ice-cream that I like as much as Ben and Jerry's so I have small amounts of that.
Also: I drink wine every night and coffee for breakfast with Coffee-mate.

Well, it didn't take me long to diagnose her problems. The first two are easy to spot. Number one: Sorry, guys, but pork and fish ain't plant-strong. As we saw in chapter 1, *all* animal-based foods are weak foods, and your body doesn't deserve anything less than the strongest health-promoting foods out there.

Number two: Too many of Pamela's food choices are processed—I'm looking at you, veggie dogs and Amy's frozen entrées!

Third, everyone say it with me: *Oil is not a health food!* Oil is a weak, refined, processed, calorie-laden, nutrient-vacant, unhealthy pile of unnecessary fat.

But beyond the obvious problems, see if you can spot the main reason Pamela isn't losing any weight. Hint: It's not so much about what she's eating. Nope. You see, Pamela has a drinking problem. And no, I don't mean the old-fashioned kind of boozy hazes. I mean the kind that somehow talks you into drinking something around the order of 1,800 calories a day. For example, in Pamela's case, each of those three smoothies she drinks on a daily basis contains approximately 450 calories. Add those calories in with those in the wine and the coffee creamer, and it's no wonder Pamela isn't losing weight!

Here's an example that really drives home this point: I met an elderly gentleman named Darren who told me he was eating only superclean, calorie-light, nutrient-dense, plant-based foods, and yet he still couldn't lose that extra abdominal flab. I asked him to tell me what a typical day of food looked like. He didn't have to get past his "breakfast" before I realized the problem.

Darren, like Pamela, had a drinking problem! He began each day with a cocktail of what he deemed "a nutrient-dense explosion" of twenty-one "super" ingredients that he guzzled to begin his day. The twenty-one ingredients were kale, parsley, cilantro, celery, cucumber, spinach, romaine lettuce, mint, 1 cup frozen strawberries, 1 banana, ½ cup frozen blueberries, one huge handful of fresh cranberries, 1 tablespoon flaxseed oil, 1 tablespoon ground flaxseeds, 1 tablespoon sunflower seeds, 1 tablespoon chia seeds, 1 tablespoon hemp seeds, 1 teaspoon cinnamon, 1 teaspoon turmeric, ¼ teaspoon pepper, and a pinch of cayenne pepper! Absolutely amazing! If you add up all the calories in that one "nutrient explosion," you get a caloric explosion in the neighborhood of 750 to 850 calories while not feeling remotely full. I will explain in great detail why Darren, although well intentioned, was unknowingly sabotaging himself at 7:30 a.m. each and every day.

We talked about eating only whole foods in chapter 2. Well, the same goes for your beverages, too—even if they're made of plants. Squeezing a bunch of oranges into a glass might seem like it would make for a healthy beverage, but actually you're turning yourself into a human food processor. You're taking six whole oranges, tossing out the fiber as well as vital nutrients, and then pulverizing them into a drink.

Try eating six whole oranges in one sitting. It's not easy—I'll bet you'll start to feel full after just two. With OJ, you're essentially extracting the sugar and throwing out the rest of the good stuff. One big glass of it can be 300 calories' worth of liquid sugar. And you're hardly full afterward: For most people, OJ is what they drink *while* they're eating their breakfast, not instead of it. In fact, when I was a firefighter, whenever we were responding to a diabetic emergency, our drink of choice to rapidly raise the patient's blood sugar levels was a stiff glass of OJ. Not Coke, not Pepsi, but good old-fashioned sugary OJ.

The truth is, I get dizzy when I think how many calories most people drink on a regular basis. Coffee with creamers and sugars, sweetened milks, orange or apple juices, sugary-sweet smoothies, juices in every color of the rainbow, sodas, Red Bulls, Frappuccinos, wine, beer . . . the list is endless. One hundred calories here, 300 calories there, and the next thing you know, you're gaining, not losing, weight—and you don't realize it's all those liquids that are to blame.

Let's start with the worst offenders: sugary beverages. Your typical 20-ounce soda contains up to 18 teaspoons of sugar and about 240 calories. You can down that sucker in less than five minutes and you won't feel any less hungry. In fact, all that sugar will make you feel more hungry. For example, in one study out of the University of Southern California, researchers hooked up 24 men and women to brain scanners and proved that drinking sugar-sweetened beverages stimulated regions of the brain that trigger food cravings.

Now, what if you had 240 calories' worth of kale? You'd have to eat more than a pound of the Queen of Greens in order to pack in 240 calories. You'd also be getting about 18 grams of fiber, 21 grams of protein, and 2,400 milligrams of potassium. You'd get nearly 308 percent of your vitamin A intake and 100 percent of vitamin B_6. And you'd be so stuffed, you wouldn't be hungry for a long time.

All that added sugar doesn't just make you fat. It can lead you into the arms of the grim reaper. A recent Tufts University analysis found that sugary drinks are responsible for 184,000 deaths globally each year, including 25,000 in the United States alone.

According to the latest Harvard University figures, in the 1970s sugary drinks represented about 4 percent of Americans' calorie intake. Today it's closer to 10 percent. Teens are racking up more calories from soda and sports drinks than from any other source. Those who drink one to two cans of soda per day have a 26 percent greater risk of developing type 2 diabetes. Meanwhile, a study published in the journal *Circulation* following 40,000 men for twenty years found that men consuming a can of soda per day had a 20 percent higher risk of having a heart attack than men who rarely had soda. And a twenty-two-year study of 80,000 women published in the *Journal of the American Medical Association* found that a can of soda per day led to a 75 percent higher risk of gout. The latest word on the street is that kids are now taking in more calories from sodas, fruit juices, smoothies, and cow secretions than they do from chewing real food.

But my problem isn't so much with sugary sodas. They're horrible for your health, but almost everyone knows that already. Indeed, a government study found that daily soda consumption in the United States fell by 20 percent between 2007 and 2013. The more insidious problems are the calorie-rich drinks that people *think* are good for us. For instance, did you know that fruit juice can be just as unhealthy as soda? A 12-ounce can of Coke has about 140 calories and 40 grams of sugar, while a 12-ounce serving of apple juice has 165 calories and 39 grams of sugar.

A new study out of the University of Connecticut found that while most parents understand that soda is bad for their kids, they mistakenly believe that other sugar-sweetened beverages, such as fruit drinks, sports drinks, and flavored waters, are *good* for them. Eighty percent regularly gave their kids fruit drinks like SunnyD or Capri Sun, and half of parents assumed that flavored waters were perfectly healthy. Maybe this has something to do with the more than $3 billion spent annually by beverage companies on marketing their products?

But there's good news: I'm going to give you a stupidly easy rule to figure out which beverages are good and which are bad. It's simple, simple, simple. Are you ready?

DON'T DRINK YOUR CALORIES

That's it. That's the rule. Don't drink your calories. Take a look at the nutrition label: If it has calories, don't let it near your lips during the next seven days.

I'll bet you didn't realize just how fast the calories add up. Let's try walking through a single day. A little morning java isn't so bad… except when you splash in the sugar and creamer. Then you have an innocent glass of OJ. It isn't even 9:00 a.m., and you've already drunk 250 calories—about the same as a medium-size bagel, but without filling you up. Next you have that lunchtime Jamba Juice smoothie. This tasty little sugar bomb packs in another 550 calories. Maybe an afternoon pick-me-up Coke after that endless meeting? That's 240 calories, followed by a 100-calorie glass of chocolate milk after the gym and a 125-calorie glass of red wine during dinner. Sounds reasonable, right? Well, you've just binged on nearly 1,300 calories. That's much more than half of your entire calorie allotment for the day, and we're not even counting the food you actually eat yet! When you drink your calories, your brain and your stomach don't register them as actual calories. You eat the same amount of food during the day on top of any liquid calories you've poured down the old hatch.

By drinking that smoothie, you're pulling a fast one on your stomach—it's the equivalent of eating a Big Mac, and your body is none the wiser. As a result, you end up drinking tons of calories alongside whatever food you're eating. Think about it—when was the last time something you drank made you less hungry? Fruit juices are made by grinding and pulverizing whole-food fiber into a million tiny pieces—to the point where it's no longer effective at triggering the stretch receptors in your stomach to alert your brain that you're full. When you eat whole fruits and veggies, on the other hand, the fiber in the food you swallow triggers these stretch receptors, which in turn tell your brain to stop eating. (We will talk about this principle in more detail in chapter 4: "Why We Care about Calorie Density.")

In addition, liquid calories cause a sudden spike in your blood sugar levels, which then leads to a spike in insulin levels, which causes your liver to boost levels of cholesterol and triglycerides. Think of your liver as a gas tank: It can process only so much sugar at a time. Drinking a soda or a glass of OJ is like trying to dump 50 gallons of gas into a 25-gallon tank—a bunch is going to spill out. Some of that sugar is converted into energy for your muscles and cells, but the rest—as much as 30 percent—spews out of that gas tank and is converted into pure fat as a last resort. That means fat in your blood (which leads to high cholesterol and triglyceride levels) and unsightly body fat in your butt, thighs, and belly. Constantly inundating your system with blood sugar spikes can lead to inflammation and heart disease by raising your C-reactive protein levels—a key marker of inflammation in your body—not to mention causing weight gain and insulin resistance by adding body fat.

A 2013 Harvard University analysis involving three separate studies and 187,000 participants found that greater juice consumption was associated with a high risk of diabetes. Conversely, people who ate three servings a week of blueberries—not blueberry juice!—had a 26 percent reduced chance of developing diabetes. Grapes? Twelve percent reduced risk. Pears? Seven percent. But drinking fruit juice regularly? That was associated with an 8 percent *increased* risk of developing diabetes. Meanwhile, merely replacing three servings per week of fruit juice with whole blueberries could cut your diabetes risk by 33 percent.

When you eat the whole fruit, the sugar is converted to energy like a big log in a slow-burning fire—that is, steady and controlled. Your liver can take its time since whole fruits are digested over time, not all at once. There is no sugar spike, and your body never has to convert excess sugar into fat.

Instead of harming your body, whole fruit makes it stronger. An American Cancer Society study of nearly 100,000 people found that those who ate the most whole berries were much less likely to die of cardiovascular disease compared to people who ate the least. Another analysis of nine separate studies published in the *Journal of Nutrition* found that your risk of heart disease decreases by 7 percent for each daily serving of fruit. On the flip side, researchers reported in the journal *Appetite* that "the daily use of fruit juice may increase central blood pressures, which are known to be associated with cardiovascular disease risk and cognitive impairment."

Go find an apple and take a nice healthy bite. This initial bite marks the beginning of a long period of digestion. Your salivary glands immediately release an enzyme called salivary amylase, which helps to keep the sugar bonded to the apple's carbohydrates. When you swallow, the intact fruit passes into your stomach and small intestines, where another enzyme, pancreatic amylase, methodically breaks down the carbohydrates. Then, enzymes lining your intestines complete the job by making the carbs tiny enough to be absorbed into your bloodstream. It's a long, controlled process perfected by millions of years of evolution to ensure that the sugar in fruit does not hit you all at once and mess with your biochemistry. Control your blood sugar levels during the Engine 2 Rescue by chewing your apples instead of drinking them. At the end of one Rescue Week last year, we witnessed an average drop in fasting blood sugar levels of 5 mg/dl, with some people's dropping as much as 57 mg/dl. Yours can, too!

> I practiced chewing a lot more, really pulverizing each bite. Slowing down and chewing allowed me to eat and realize when I was full, rather than plowing through the entire giant salad and then feeling overstuffed and bloated.
> —Mark Longfellow, age 49, software test analyst

The fiber in your apple helps slow down digestion, control the release of sugar into the blood, and make you feel full and satiated. But you need to eat the whole fruit to reap the benefits. For example, a glass of apple juice contains a paltry 0.5 gram of fiber, while a whole apple contains up to 5 grams (the skin alone contains nearly 2 grams). All that missing fiber is why drinking lots of juice is associated with weight gain and diabetes, while eating lots of whole fruit is not.

Here's a great case in point: In one South African study, seventeen people were asked to eat twenty servings of fruit every single day for months on end. Not only did they not turn into a giant blueberry like Violet Beauregarde in *Willy Wonka*, but, despite eating all that fruit—the sugar equivalent of downing eight cans of soda per day—six months into the study the researchers reported that they had found no adverse effects on the subjects' body weight, blood pressure, insulin, cholesterol, or triglyceride levels. A very similar study found that participants eating twenty daily servings of fruit lowered their cholesterol by an average of 38 points!

The moral of the story: *eat* your fruit, don't drink it.

Savor That Skin!

An apple a day keeps the oncologist away. A study published in the *Annals of Oncology* found that women who eat apples daily have 24 percent lower odds of developing breast cancer compared to women who don't bother with that daily apple. That's on top of lower odds of ovarian cancer, laryngeal cancer, and colorectal cancer.

The reason seems to be that the apple's antioxidants—those free radical– and cancer-fighting machines we talked about in chapter 1—are concentrated in its skin. In fact, the antioxidant power of the apple skin may be as much as six times greater than the apple pulp.

This isn't chemotherapy—we're just talking about apples here. Sadly, this wonderful peel doesn't get the respect it deserves: In just the country of Chile alone, apple producers toss away *9,000* tons of peels each year to make dried apple products. If one mere apple can reduce your risk of cancer, imagine what 9,000 tons of apple peels could do!

Another problem is that your body does not compensate for the calories it drinks. If you eat a whole baked potato for lunch, you're going to feel full and eat less food throughout the rest of the day. You have to work hard to chew and swallow those calories, and both your mind and your stomach will tell you to ease off the food for a while once you've had enough.

Proof comes from a 2009 study in the *Journal of the American Dietetic Association*: Twenty normal-weight and 20 obese adults were given 300 calories of either whole apples, applesauce, or apple juice. The study concluded: "Whether consumed with a meal or alone as a snack, the beverage elicited the weakest appetitive response, the solid food form elicited the strongest appetitive response and the semisolid response was intermediate." In other words, *drinking* the same amount of calories found in the whole food does not fill you up nearly as well.

Juicing

One of the biggest dietary trends going on now is juicing, which its proponents say increases your consumption of vital nutrients. Is this true? Can you juice your way to good health?

The quick answer is: No!

(Do you remember Darren at the beginning of this chapter?)

To debunk the juicing fad, I asked my father why he's so averse to people drinking not only their calories, but in particular the newfangled kale/spinach/beet and other color-of-the-rainbow vegetable and fruit juices. He says it's important to chew your greens if you want to maximize the abilities of these amazing leafy cruciferous vegetables to impact nitric-oxide production by your endothelial cells (the cells lining your arteries). Nitric oxide (NO) is a critical chemical compound in your body that is released by the cells in your arteries, signaling muscle fibers in your cell walls to relax and allow more blood to flow.

The ability of your endothelial cells to pump out nitric oxide is a direct marker of the health of your vessels. The more your endothelial cells produce NO, the better their ability to keep the inner lining of your vessels smooth like Teflon instead of rough like Velcro. Typically, when we are fifty, our bodies are producing 50 percent less nitric oxide than when we were twenty-five.

The good news is that there is a plant-friendly way to compensate for this diminished endothelial nitric oxide production—chew your leafy greens!

When you chew—and *only* by chewing—your leafy greens (kale, Swiss chard, spinach, arugula, beet greens, Napa cabbage, etc.), the anaerobic bacteria residing in the crevices and grooves of your tongue reduce the nitrates in these leafy greens. Then, when you swallow these nitrites, the gastric acid in your stomach further reduces them to nitric oxide, which enters and combines with your existing nitric oxide pool.

Some nitrites in your stomach do not get reduced into nitric oxide, however. Instead, they continue farther downstream into your gut and eventually are reabsorbed into the bloodstream. Your circulatory system carries these auxiliary nitrites back to your salivary glands where they will be concentrated ten- to twentyfold. As you chew more food, your own saliva pours the nitrites into your mouth and the whole process begins again. The nitrites will be further reduced by the gastric acid in your stomach into more nitric oxide. *Bam!* It's a nitric-oxide party in your mouth, your gut, and in your endothelial cells!

This is an extremely delicate process honed by thousands of years of evolution. When you drink your green smoothies and juices, you bypass this synergistic and wonderful system and miss out on one of the most powerful holistic reasons for including green leafies in your diet. This is why I want you eating green leafy vegetables as often as possible during the Seven-Day Rescue.

In addition, another big reason we don't like smoothies and juicing is because when you throw fruits and vegetables into that mixer, you break the fiber into a jillion little pieces, separating it from the fructose, which is absorbed like a rocket and subsequently hits the liver, impairs the protein, and injures your vital endothelial cells, making it more difficult for blood to flow.

So if you drink your calories, you actively hurt your body. If you eat your calories, you actively make your body healthier (as long as you're choosing plant-strong food!).

Here it is, plain and simple: Chew your food. You know, like how your parents taught you in the high chair. Breast-feeding (or bottle-feeding) as an infant should be the only point in life that we drink our calories. Instead, humans are the only mammals that continue to drink their calories into adulthood. Chewing food is one of the first things we ever learn. Now everyone is forgetting how to do it!

Don't Drink Your Fake Calories!

What about diet sodas? It's true they don't have any calories. Are they safe to drink?

No!

First, artificial sweeteners are not healthy! The most popular, aspartame (Equal), which is used in many diet sodas, is associated with an increased risk of depression. More recently, a report published in the *Southern Medical Journal* linked the sweetener to hypertension, and there have also been case reports of aspartame-induced brain conditions including pseudo-tumor cerebri, a condition in which the pressure inside your skull increases dangerously. Meanwhile, a study published in the *AAOHN Journal* noted that sucralose (Splenda) has been linked to migraine headaches, and stevia was potentially linked to DNA damage in a study published by the journal *Mutagenesis*.

Moreover, drinking fake sugar can cause you to eat more food overall. For example, a study in the *American Journal of Clinical Nutrition* revealed that choosing artificially sweetened beverages encourages people (subconsciously) to overeat later in the day. *Hey,* the underlying thinking goes, *if that Diet Coke cost me zero calories, I must have room for that Snickers bar.* In addition, artificially sweetened beverages trigger ancient evolutionary impulses to eat as much sweet food as possible—after all, our ancestors might have gone months before seeing another mouthwatering berry patch. Without the appetite-suppressing effects of actual fruit, the more artificially sweetened drinks you have, the more you crave food.

Bingeing on sweeteners has the effect of essentially making you a Diet Coke junkie. Everyone knows that guy in the office who downs six or seven Diet Cokes a day. It's not because he likes the sweet—it's because he *needs* the sweet. By regularly drinking sugar- and artificially sweetened drinks, he is programming his taste buds to demand sweetness at every meal. (And if there isn't any fake sugar around, that junkie is going to go for the real stuff: pie, cookies, candy.)

Stay away from artificial sweeteners. They may contain zero calories, but the harmful effects on your body are anything but zero.

Alcohol

Let's talk a little about alcohol. Don't worry, I'm not going to give you a Nancy Reagan chat about morals here. After a great shift at the firehouse or on special occasions, I've had a couple of relaxing cold ones. My issue with alcohol has less to do with the way it affects your mind and more to do with how it affects the rest of your body.

Like soda and fruit juice, alcoholic drinks are entirely empty calories. One jigger of whiskey contains 105 calories, a pint of beer can have close to 200 calories, and that after-work gin and tonic is another 200 calories. But the problem with liquor extends beyond the calories. Alcohol inhibits your body's ability to burn fat by as much as 30 percent, and it's a known toxin to just about every organ in your body, especially your liver, brain, heart, and kidneys—important organs you want to keep around as long as possible.

Everyone knows about alcohol's effect on decision-making abilities, but it also leads to some other bad choices aside from drinking and driving. You down lots of booze and suddenly you get the munchies. Why not have a double-cheese pizza and a carton of wings and maybe a cupcake or two? Before long, those 300 empty alcohol calories lead to 1,500 empty food calories.

Still another reason I don't encourage a lot of alcohol: There are no nutrition labels on those bottles. Most people have no idea how many calories they're taking in with each sip, shot, or gulp. The fact is, a bottle of wine a week will add about 10 pounds' worth of calories a year, as will a bottle of beer every night. And that's just one bottle!

While half of all alcohol-related deaths are related to drunk driving and other accidents, the other half are due to liver disease. Drinking alcohol in excess amounts leads to the inflammation and accumulation of fat in the liver, a condition called fatty liver disease. The CDC notes that excess drinking means more than two drinks a day for men or one drink a day for women, but the Cleveland Clinic points out that up to 40 percent of people with more modest alcohol intake can also develop fatty deposits in their livers. The bottom line is that any amount of alcohol can cause liver inflammation.

So what's the big deal? We've all got some flab in our bellies and thighs; what's a little more in the liver? Well, heavy drinking can result in a fatty liver in as little as three weeks. Over time, as you continue to drink, repeated inflammation and fat deposits can lead to a condition called alcohol-induced hepatitis and, eventually, cirrhosis, an irreversible scarring of the liver. Scar tissue cannot do what healthy liver tissue can: make proteins, fight infections, clean the blood. Only by cutting out alcohol entirely can you stop alcohol-induced liver disease before it's too late. Nothing can make scarred tissue go away, but removing alcohol from the equation can prevent liver scarring from getting worse.

There's more bad news: Alcohol consumption has been linked to cancer. In fact, in its 2011 "Report on Carcinogens," the US Department of Health and Human Services listed alcohol as a known human carcinogen, and the World Health Organization upgraded its categorization of alcohol to a definitive human breast carcinogen. When you drink, your body metabolizes the ethanol in drinks into acetaldehyde, a toxic chemical that can damage cell DNA, possibly leading to cancerous mutations. In addition, alcohol intake can give rise to free radicals, those unstable molecules that stampede through your bloodstream, smashing into other cells and causing cancerous mutations by scrambling their DNA.

The American Cancer Society reports that women who consume

between two and five drinks daily are 1.5 times more likely to develop breast cancer than women who don't drink. Until recently, though, very little research had been done on light drinking. Does just one drink a day really increase your risk of breast cancer?

Yes, it does.

In 2013, Italian researchers decided to gather all the best studies comparing light drinkers to abstainers. The meta-analysis consisted of more than two hundred separate studies that comprised 92,000 light drinkers (one drink a day or less) and 60,000 nondrinkers. Overall, the researchers estimated that nearly 5,000 breast cancer deaths per year worldwide are attributable to light drinking (not to mention 24,000 deaths from esophageal cancer). Yes, this means that 5,000 deaths every year are caused by something as innocent as a little after-work chardonnay. Not long after these results were published, the medical journal *Breast* published an editorial stating that "women who consume alcohol chronically have an increased risk for breast cancer that is dose dependent but without threshold." In other words, there is no level of alcohol consumption that doesn't raise breast cancer risk.

And sorry, guys, but the same appears true for prostate cancer. A study published in the journal *Cancer* following 10,000 men found that those who drank heavily were more than twice as likely to develop very aggressive prostate cancer compared to men who drank less often. But the risk remains even among nonheavy drinkers: a group of Harvard University researchers discovered "a positive association between moderate alcohol consumption and the risk of prostate cancer" in their study of more than 7,500 men.

If you don't take it from me, take it from the World Health Organization: No amount of alcohol is safe. Let the Seven-Day Rescue be your chance to remove alcohol for a week, and in the process clean up your liver and other vital organs.

The Milk Perversion

Milk is liquid meat. It's as simple as that. Here's what I mean: A teeny-tiny 1-ounce serving of beef has about 3.2 grams of saturated fat and 22 mg of cholesterol. A mere cup of 2 percent milk has 3.1 grams of saturated fat and 20 mg of cholesterol. You drop a hunk of meat in the blender and you're effectively drinking the same chronic-disease-causing cocktail.

Not only are humans the only mammals on earth who drink their calories into adulthood, we're the only mammals who drink milk from *other* mammals. Have you ever thought about the fact that milk helps calves grow from their 60-pound birth weight to 1,200 pounds in just one year? Cow's milk has been designed by thousands of years of evolution to pack two pounds a day onto a growing calf—that's forty times the growth rate of humans. For the calves, this extremely high-fat liquid is healthy. Do you see human babies growing to be 1,200 pounds after a year on their mothers' milk? Of course not! That's because humans are meant to drink human milk and cows are meant to drink cow's milk. As the renowned physician and author Michael Klaper says, "Cow's milk is baby calf growth fluid. It's loaded with IGF-1, hormones, estrogens, animal protein, and saturated fat. Run, don't walk, away from it!"

Nonetheless, although our kids aren't growing up to be as big as Texas longhorns, we are seeing them grow fatter than ever before. In fact, over the last few decades the number of American children classified as overweight has increased by more than 100 percent. More than one-third of all children and teens are now overweight or obese. And studies routinely show that 75 to 80 percent of kids who are obese will remain that way as adults. Kids who are overweight as teenagers may have twice the risk of dying from heart disease in adulthood, not to mention being at a much higher risk of developing other chronic diseases such as certain cancers, arthritis, and gout. The problem has become so acute that we're seeing type 2 diabetes in children as young as eight. And a fifteen-year study published in the journal *Diabetes* found that such early diabetes diagnoses have destructive consequences later in life, including high incidences of amputation, blindness, kidney failure, heart disease, and premature death.

Yeah, but what does this have to do with milk? What, those little innocent-looking cartons of milk with cute pictures of happy cows might be responsible for this?

You better believe it. The problem has a lot to do with protein in cow's milk. Did you know that the protein levels in human breast milk are the lowest among all mammals? It should be no surprise that the protein in cow's milk, which is designed to pack pounds onto a much larger creature, ends up doing the same to our kids. A study published in the *Journal of Nutrition* found that teens exposed to dairy milk—even skim milk—suffered from significant increases in body mass index

(BMI) and waist circumference. Another study published in the journal *Archives of Pediatrics and Adolescent Medicine*, which followed more than 12,000 children nationwide, found that kids consuming more than three servings of dairy milk daily were 35 percent more likely to become overweight compared to kids who drank less.

The problems only seem to get worse the earlier kids start drinking cow's milk. For example, a study published in *PLOS ONE*, the journal of the Public Library of Science, discovered that high milk intake early in life is associated with girls' experiencing their first period much earlier than normal. A landmark study in the *New England Journal of Medicine* reported that cow's milk can be directly blamed for childhood constipation as well as an extremely painful condition known as anal fissure. In two-thirds of the children studied, the constipation and fissures were cured entirely by replacing cow's milk with soy milk, while none of the children who continued to drink cow's milk saw an improvement in their health. This confirms why other studies have suggested that kids who drink a cup of milk a day may have eight times the odds of developing fissures, and how 80 percent of childhood constipation can be cured by simply removing dairy milk from the diet.

So instead of asking, "Got milk?" maybe they should ask, "Got constipation?"

Milk and Acne

Tell you what: if you won't stop drinking milk to improve your body, maybe you will stop drinking milk to improve your face.

Harvard University researchers decided to follow 6,000 girls ages nine to fifteen for a few years to find out if there was a link between milk consumption and diet. Sure enough, they discovered a "positive association between intake of milk and acne." The same was found for teenage boys in a subsequent study. Choosing skim milk doesn't help—studies have found that concentrations of steroid sex hormones, which are thought to promote the acne, are highest in skim milk.

If you travel abroad, you might notice that people in other nations often have smoother skin. That's because acne, which afflicts up to 95 percent of American teens and half of adults under forty, is almost exclusively a Western phenomenon—much like dairy milk consumption. For example, in a study published in the *Archives of Dermatology*, researchers following 1,200 predominantly plant-based and dairy-milk-free people in New Guinea and remote regions of Paraguay could not diagnose a single pimple during a period of more than two years.

Meanwhile, don't believe any of the dairy industry's claims about the so-called bone-strengthening benefits of milk. In fact, quite the opposite is true. When consumed, animal products create an acidic environment in the bloodstream. In response, the body leaches calcium from the bones in order to neutralize the acid. Consumption of dairy products, especially those labeled as low-fat or nonfat (meaning they have a higher percentage of protein), can therefore lead to *lower* levels of calcium in the body. Indeed, one set of studies published by the *BMJ* that analyzed 100,000 people for two decades suggested that milk can actually *increase* the rates of bone and hip fractures, which might explain why some of the highest rates of osteoporosis are found in the countries with the highest rates of dairy consumption. Americans consume more calcium from dairy products than any other nation, and yet we have the highest incidence of osteoporosis. Something must give, and it turns out to be your bones.

It seems the negative effects of milk on the body only become worse with age. Think about this for a moment: Milk is specifically designed to help a baby—whether it's a calf or a human—grow as fast as possible. That's why milk is packed with growth hormones and sex steroid hormones like estrogen. When you've stopped growing, however, these hormones help grow cancerous tumors instead of bones.

The association between milk and prostate cancer was proved by a study published in the journal *Nutrition and Cancer*. Researchers dripped milk directly onto prostate cancer cells in a laboratory, which had the effect of turbocharging the cancer progression in each of the fourteen experiments they performed, fueling the cancer growth rate by more than 30 percent. Moreover, a 2015 meta-analysis published in the *American Journal of Clinical Nutrition* concluded that a high intake of dairy products, including whole and low-fat milk, appears to increase a man's risk of prostate cancer.

The research suggests milk can cause problems even before birth— "Women attempting conception should avoid milk and dairy products," concluded one study in the *Journal of Reproductive Medicine*. Why? Because potentially unsafe complications such as twinning may occur, which may explain why women who eat entirely plant-based diets give birth to twins at just one-fifth the rate of omnivores.

All the evidence screams one simple point: Dairy milk is unsafe at any age. Leave cow's milk for baby cows. Repeat after me, "No moo milk here!"

Box: Monkey Milk Anyone?

Firefighters work twenty-four hours straight and then have forty-eight hours off. My team was the C shift— while we were gone from the station, the A shift took over, and after them, the B shift. That meant we had patches of downtime, and we were used to coming up with new ways to keep busy, which usually involved competitions: everything from marathon Ping-Pong tournaments to racing up the fire pole hand over hand.

But one evening three of us—James Rae (aka JR), Josh Miller, and I—were sitting on the firehouse porch talking about health and cholesterol levels. Soon enough, we'd made a bet to see whose cholesterol level was lowest, and the next day we drove to a lab and got tested.

When we got the results, JR—whose cholesterol level was a whopping 344 mg/dl—lost the bet by a landside. This got us worried, because all of the males in the Rae family have had a knack for falling over dead from heart attacks at a young age. We put JR on a healthful, plant-strong diet, and soon the rest of the crew was eating plant-based meals, too—and that's how Engine 2 became Austin's famous plant-eating fire brigade.

Not everyone was happy about this. Many firefighters feel very strongly about their meat. And so we plant eaters at Engine 2 found ourselves in a lot of arguments with the meat eaters at other firehouses—which I am sure we won.

Of course, making fun bets and arguing aren't the only ways firefighters pass time. They also like to engage in worms. Worms are not dietary, nor are they animals. In the Austin Fire Department, a "worm" is a type of practical joke. It's called a worm because the goal is to burrow down and get under someone's skin. And worms were played there, all the time, by everyone.

For example, not long after Engine 2 got a great deal of publicity for our plant-strong lifestyle, the meat-loving guys at Station 4 decided that a worm was necessary to put us in our place. So one very hot afternoon, while we were out flowing hydrants in our territory, they drove over to Station 2, snuck into our bathrooms, and carefully placed crushed-up beef bouillon cubes in the showerheads. When we plant eaters came back in to clean up, we were soon bathing in nothing but meat juice. Smelly, sticky, yucky meat drippings!

This did not make us happy! Not. One. Bit. This worm successfully got on our skin and under it!

As you can guess, one good worm deserves another. So a few weeks later, I traveled over to Station 4 to fill in for an absent firefighter. The next morning, as we were eating breakfast, the guys started talking about health and nutrition (as we always do at some point when I'm around).

One of the guys was gulping whole milk straight out of a gallon jug and asked, "Rip, is this good for me?"

"Nope," I said. I told him that humans are the only mammals that drink another mammal's milk, and I added that cow's milk was the perfect food for a heifer, changing her from a 60-pound baby to a 1,000-pound adult, but since humans aren't descended from bovines, it would be much better for him to drink monkey milk. It has, I said, a much better blend of protein, carbohydrates, and fat.

"Monkey milk!" one of the guys said. "That sounds kind of weird, but I guess it makes sense! Is it for sale some place in Austin?"

"Well, it's funny you ask," I said. "Whole Foods Market just started carrying it. I think it comes in sweetened and unsweetened, and in chocolate and vanilla as well."

The guys got very excited. They loved milk, and now they were going to be drinking the best milk possible, monkey milk!

We got off shift at noon, and at 1:30 p.m. I got a phone call from one of the guys. He was out shopping at the Whole Foods at Sixth Street and Lamar Boulevard, searching for monkey milk. "Hey, Rip," he said, "I'm at the store but I can't find the monkey's milk. Do you know what section it's in?"

Worming works best when you can stretch it out. "It's definitely in the dairy section, but they're probably out of it since it's such a novelty item," I said. "But I bet they have it at the Gateway Center Whole Foods store."

"Okay," he said. "By the way, is there a brand?"

"Sure," I said. "You want to buy COB."

"COB?"

"Yes. It stands for chimpanzee, orangutan, and baboon."

"Got it, Rip. This is going to be so cool…to drink monkey's milk!"

So off he went to the Gateway store, which was ten miles away. About forty-five minutes later, I got another call.

"Hey, Rip, so not only have I been up and down the dairy aisle twice, but I've also asked three different Whole Foods employees if they know anything about this new alternative milk product called COB or monkey's milk, and they're looking at me as if I have three heads!"

Then I waited, taking the perfect pause. "Remember the beef bouillon cubes in the showers at Station 2? Well, this is payback, you dirty dog!" And then I made a series of monkey noises and together we laughed long and hard!

SO WHAT THE HECK *SHOULD* YOU DRINK?

Repeat it with me again: don't drink your calories! What's left to drink, then? Here's a hint: it's colorless, odorless, transparent, and it's the most important liquid in the entire universe.

I'm talking about water. Not vitamin water, coconut water, fruit water, or any other flavored calorie-infested junk. Just plain old water. Not drinking enough of it has been linked to bone fractures, heart disease, lung conditions, kidney stones, colon cancer, urinary tract infections, constipation, cavities, compromised immune systems…I could go on for pages and pages. Don't want bladder cancer? Drink more water. A Harvard University study of nearly 50,000 men found that the risk of this painful and deadly condition drops by 7 percent for every cup of water you drink daily. Don't want a heart attack? Drink more water. The Adventist Health Study, which followed more than 20,000 people, determined that people who drink five or more glasses of water per day have half the risk of dying from heart disease compared to people who drink two glasses or less.

Drink water and drink it often. The beauty of a plant-strong diet is that so many of our favorite foods are already naturally brimming with luscious water. Load up on strawberries, for instance—they're 92 percent water, which, along with their high fiber content, is why they're so satiating. A serving of strawberries supplies you with 136 grams of water. Meanwhile, a single apple packs in 116 grams of water, and a small serving of broccoli delivers 40 grams of water.

In addition to lots of yummy fruits and veggies, you should drink a minimum of six cups of water per day—up to eleven cups if you exercise frequently. Remember, the human body is 70 percent water, and you need to keep it that way! Most fruits and veggies are between 80 and 95 percent water, so when you eat healthy, you're also drinking healthy!

Don't Shrink Your Brain

Did you know that your brain is 75 percent water? If you don't drink enough water, your brain actually begins to shrink. That may explain why your mental performance diminishes along with your athletic performance if you haven't been guzzling enough of the good stuff. So keep chugging that water to keep your brain chugging along at peak performance. Cold water is best—it gets absorbed into your bloodstream 20 percent faster than warm water.

One of the first signs of dehydration can be a headache. Think of it as your brain's way of telling you: "Hey, man! I'm shrinking up here. Drink some water!"

Yeah, you say, you hear all this...but you wonder, doesn't water get a little, well, boring after a while? Myself, I don't think so, but sure, there are some great plant-strong ways to add a little flavor to life's elixir. Take a lemon wedge, lime wedge, orange wedge, or slices of cucumber and add them to your glass of water for a nice flavor boost. Try making spa water by putting fruit, cucumber, lemon, or lime slices in a pitcher of water overnight in the fridge. Or, why not combine water with one of the most antioxidant-packed, cancer-fighting plants out there?

Yup, I'm talking about tea. Black, green, and white tea all come from the same thing: the tea plant, maybe one of the most badass plants on the face of the planet. How? Let's start with cancer prevention. Researchers have noticed recently that women living in Asia are up to five times less likely to be diagnosed with breast cancer compared to American women, and the leading theory is that in addition to eating more plants, their advantage is due to the consumption of green tea, a staple of many Asian diets. Green tea, made from unfermented leaves of the tea plant, has been associated with as much as a 30 percent reduced risk of breast cancer.

Tea leaves are extremely rich in antioxidants, especially polyphenols, which act like seek-and-destroy missiles for free radicals in your bloodstream. In addition to breast cancer prevention, drinking tea has been found to protect against ovarian and endometrial cancer, diabetes, and seasonal allergies; to help lower your cholesterol, blood pressure, blood sugar, and body fat; and to help protect your brain against stroke and dementia.

But the party doesn't stop with the almighty tea plant. Herbal tea—which comes from any plant *other* than the tea plant—can also have amazing health benefits. Take hibiscus tea, for example. It's derived from the beautiful hibiscus flower and has a nice tart cranberry flavor. Don't let that innocent-looking little flower fool you, though: A study published in the *Nutrition Journal* ranked hibiscus tea number one in total antioxidant content of all 280 beverages examined. In addition to anticancer effects, hibiscus tea has been found to be extremely effective against high blood pressure. Another study out of Tufts University found that simply drinking a cup of hibiscus tea at each meal could drop systolic blood pressure significantly. Moreover, two cups of hibiscus tea in the morning was found to be just as effective at lowering blood pressure as a twice-daily 25 mg dose of the leading antihypertensive drug captopril—and, of course, without all the nasty side effects. (Tip: The wondrous health benefits of tea can be wiped out when you sweeten it with sugar or artificial sweeteners. So keep your tea clean!)

When you drink your calories instead of eating them, you don't take pleasure in your food. You can down a Cherry Coke in twenty seconds. How boring. Instead, take twenty minutes and savor a wonderful plate of Lazy Days Tostados (page 252). Let the next seven days be your opportunity to stop any bad drinking habits you may have developed over the years. Instead of drinking your calories, eat your calories! It's a lot more fun, nutritious, and natural.

I felt very satiated eating these foods. I would make a large "bowl" and think I'm still going to be hungry but halfway through I'd feel full. I learned to eat my greens first or I'd be too full to eat them.

My daughter saw me walking upstairs for bed (had my nightgown on) and she said "Momma, I can really tell you've lost weight in that!" I felt very proud!
—Jackie Clark, age 40, nurse

4

Why We Care about Calorie Density

"Eat food. Not too much. Mostly plants."

It's a catchy maxim. It's simple. On first glance it makes sense. The phrase was coined by Michael Pollan, renowned professor, journalist, and best-selling author of *In Defense of Food*, who was instructing his readers on how to navigate the "incredibly complicated and confusing question of what we humans should eat in order to be maximally healthy."

The only thing is, I don't agree with Michael. I suspect he does us all a disservice by watering down the principles of sound nutrition with comforting rhetoric.

The first principle seems easy, right? "Eat food." Well, okay—if you don't eat, you die. But food can mean brown rice or brown sugar. Apples or apple pie. Shouldn't we distinguish between healthy food and unhealthy food?

What about "Not too much"? What does that mean exactly? Does feeling full mean we have eaten too much?

And what's with "Mostly plants"? Does that mean one serving of meat per meal is okay? Per day? Per week?

I respect Michael. But I'd change that first sentence to "Eat whole food," based on what we learned in chapter 2. After all, "Eat food" can mean Doritos and Big Macs, or it can mean spinach and quinoa.

Michael completely loses me with "Not too much." All this does is add fuel to the fire that you need to limit portion sizes to lose weight. Not good! I don't want to be hungry all the time. I should be full and patting my belly after every meal! I want to eat as much food as I darn well please!

And don't get me started on "Mostly plants." This really steams my clams! We already know that the eradication of 90 percent of chronic Western diseases, the reversal of climate change, the healing of the environment, and the end of animal cruelty can happen by amending that statement to "Only plants." Not *some* plants. Not *usually* plants. Not *mostly* plants. *Only* plants.

As I've written in my other books, Americans are lousy at moderation. Or rather, we're gold medalists at peddling the belief that we can eat anything and everything so long as it's "in moderation." The reality is that moderation is the enemy within that rides in waving a white flag and then mows us down with a machine gun with excuses like "This little bit can't hurt," and "Man, I've had a hard day. I deserve this." Moderation is a dangerous and insidious slippery slope that'll have you back to your old ways before you can say "Triple bacon cheeseburger with mayo."

What's up with this "moderation" obsession, anyway? Michael Jordan didn't let up after winning one NBA championship; he won six and was MVP each time. Michael Phelps wasn't content with a nice, moderate half dozen Olympic medals—he wanted an extreme number in the twenties. Secretariat didn't just win the Triple Crown; he set course records at each race and thoroughly demolished the competition.

Moderation doesn't know victory. Moderation doesn't know glory. Moderation appeals to the lowest common denominator. Moderation is the path of least resistance. It's the weak compromise. It's the ribbon for just showing up. It's true with sports and it's true with food: moderation is your Achilles' heel, and it has no place in your refrigerator.

Now is not the time for half measures. Now is the time for you to jump in with both feet and embrace an uncompromising whole-food, plant-strong lifestyle that will start you on the path to healing. It's a simple solution to a multidimensional set of problems that has you, families, cities, states, corporations, and our government scratching their heads looking for an answer. The health-care crisis afoot in this country is a veritable bloodbath that is sucking this country dry. And the warming of our planet is a veritable greenhouse nightmare that is sucking Mother Earth dry.

The most effective tool for resolving and treating both of these pressing issues is the most overlooked and underutilized tool sitting before us: whole, plant-based food. Unfortunately, most Americans are victims of what Dr. Doug Lisle, author and director of research for the TrueNorth Health Center, calls the "pleasure trap." In short, people eating low-fat, high-fiber, plant-strong diets will experience a nice range of pleasure. However, if processed and animal foods are allowed into the diet, they will quickly become preferred. We can get hooked on their huge amounts of addictive salt, sugar, and fat. We'll eventually choose French fries over whole potatoes, and we'll pick processed energy bars over fresh fruit. A recovering heroin addict can't shoot up in moderation, nor can an alcoholic sip a little chardonnay. The only solution is to cut out the problem altogether. The good news is that after you're 100 percent plant-strong for a good amount of time, you won't want to go back. You'll take one look at that artery-busting fried chicken and gag. You'll take one whiff of that chicken soup loaded with salt and wince. Meanwhile, the Triple Pepper Chipotle Chili (page 248) will make your mouth water.

I'm going to amend Michael Pollan's maxim to the following:

Eat whole food. As much as you want. Only plants.

We saw in chapter 1 why plants are the only way to go, and in chapter 2 we learned why unprocessed whole foods outmuscle processed foods. In this chapter I will explain the primary reason why changing your diet is fun and easy: You can eat as much as you want! No calorie counting or portion control! As long as you pick the right foods, you can eat until your stomach is happily full and still lose weight.

We have become so hardwired to eat less in order to lose weight that most health-conscious Americans have become serial dieters. We count calories, count points, watch portion sizes, weigh our food, and exercise until the cows come home—all without any success. Whatever weight we do lose, we gain back after we stop the diet.

Somehow we have become convinced that the bottom line when it comes to losing our ever-widening bottoms is food deprivation. And yet, even as millions of people deprive themselves of the most basic survival instinct we have as humans—eating—people are forever hopeful that an answer is out there. How else could you explain the fact that tens of thousands of diet books have been published and some people claim to have tried almost every one of them!

As I travel around the country, people bombard me with stories about how they've become "professional dieters" and are salivating for the next diet book to hit the shelves and the next essential nutrient to swear off. This is indicative of the hopeful resiliency of people who never stop searching for a solution. Unfortunately, the solution can't be found in diet books that preach extreme food deprivation. I remember when the actor Ben Foster, who played Lance Armstrong in the recent Armstrong biopic, told the media that to lose weight for his demanding role he went on an 850-calorie-per-day diet with the support of his then fiancée, Robin Wright, who joined him in an act of solidarity. Back in 2015, the *New York Times* ran a front-page article about how Jeb Bush, while running for president, lost 35 pounds by "always being hungry" following the Paleo Diet. In short, people have been conditioned to believe that losing weight means depriving themselves of food.

This practice is flawed to the core. Asking people to limit the amount of food they can eat for a day, month, or year will always eventually backfire. It's a little like asking people to limit the number of breaths they take every day. You could try, but soon you'd throw your hands up in despair because the drive to breathe, like the drive to eat, is innate and should not be restrained.

I want to shift the mind-set from *how much* we eat to *what* we eat, which will in fact make "how much" irrelevant. This has everything to do with a concept called *calorie density*.

The coolest thing about understanding calorie density principles is that you can discard all the nonsense you've heard about dieting and start over with a clean slate. It's liberating when you realize that the reason America is overweight is because our diet is heavily composed of the most calorie-rich foods on the planet. This is a no-win proposition that guarantees weight gain and the promotion of chronic disease.

A much better proposition is this one: eat mounds of food while taking in fewer calories and feeling satisfied and full!

> I think my biggest surprise during the Engine 2 Rescue Week was that I wasn't hungry. That's because I was eating so much at mealtimes. I found myself not even looking for late-night snacks by the end of the program.
> —Harry Leslie, age 58, database specialist

WHAT LEADS TO OVERCONSUMPTION?

The central theme of this chapter is that eating foods that fill you up does not have to mean you will gain weight. On the other hand, foods that do *not* fill you up often *do* make you gain weight.

Sounds paradoxical, right? Trust me, it isn't. Let's look at some of the most important factors that lead to weight gain:

Calorie-Dense Food. What does *calorie dense* mean? Well, when it comes to weight control, the overall amount of calories in a particular food is less important than its *calorie density*, that is, the amount of calories in relation to its weight. For instance, a 3.5-pound melon has just 450 calories, while 3.5 pounds of Swiss cheese has more than *6,000* calories. Because people tend to eat a certain volume of food every day, regardless of calories, one of the primary ways people gain weight is by eating too many high-calorie-dense foods such as dairy, meat, and processed junk foods, and not enough low-calorie-dense fruits, vegetables, beans, and intact whole grains such as brown rice. (See the calorie-density list on pages 97–98.)

Liquid Calories. We talked about this in chapter 3. Drinking your calories can be the equivalent of sipping a Big Mac with a straw and not feeling any less hungry. Liquid calories, which provide no sense of satiety, are a major reason why diets inevitably fail. A soda here, a smoothie there, a glass of wine later, and all of a sudden you've taken in half your daily calories, you're more hungry than ever, and you haven't even touched your food yet!

With the Engine 2 Rescue Diet we avoid this trap altogether. If your beverage has calories, don't drink it!

High-Fat Foods. Fat contains the most calories (9) per gram, so the more fat your food has, the more calories it has. It's as simple as that. Animal products are, of course, high in fat—especially the Darth Vader of fats, saturated fat—so it's no surprise that eating them leads to weight gain. Most plant foods, on the other hand, are naturally low in fat and contain only the essential amounts our bodies need to function optimally.

A review of twenty-eight studies published in the *American Journal of Clinical Nutrition* found that obesity rates have increased in countries where fat intake has risen, while obesity rates have remained low in countries consuming a traditional low-fat diet. Moreover, the analysis found that folks who switched to a low-fat diet while eating as much as they wanted were able to decrease their calorie intake by 11 to 30 percent.

Processed Bread Products. These are some of the worst offenders when it comes to promoting overeating. As we saw in chapter 2, food manufacturers remove the whole grain's bran and germ, which provide not just nutrition but also a sense of fullness. Almost all the satiety-promoting fiber, which is found only in plants, is also removed, leaving you with a loaf of empty, dense calories that won't fill you up.

Carbohydrates from refined, processed grains, such as non-whole-grain pasta, bread, and crackers, have roughly three times the caloric density of unrefined, whole-grain foods like rice, oats, and potatoes.

Dried Fruit. These impostors were once glorious fruits, but they've been tortured until almost every last drop of water has been removed and they become sugary shrivels of their former selves. We'll discuss this in more depth later, but the water content of plants is one of the primary reasons they're so satiating. You can eat three handfuls of raisins in a matter of seconds and reach for more, but I challenge you to eat thirty grapes without feeling full.

It's remarkable how many new fad diets show up every year: high-fat diets, low-fat diets, low-carb diets, high-protein diets…the list goes on and on. As with some high-performance gym routine, you might have to eat different foods on different days and account for every single calorie. There is one thing that remains constant no matter what diet you try, however: hunger. Whether it's Atkins, South Beach, Weight Watchers, or Zone, you're going to feel hungry the majority of the time due to small portions.

That's why the Engine 2 Diet blows all these weak diets out of the water. As long as you're eating the right foods, you can eat as much as you want, whenever you want. How is that possible? Read on!

In the following section I'm going to walk you through three popular methods for approaching calorie density: (1) Volumetrics, a diet plan created by Barbara Rolls, PhD, which deals with computing calorie density by looking at food labels; (2) the Hawaii Diet approach, which emphasizes an all-you-can eat buffet of low-calorie-dense foods; and (3) dietician Jeff Novick's wonderful, easy-to-understand charts for filling your plate.

Readers who are drawn to food labels and math will really like the Volumetric approach. If you hate dealing with numbers, no problem! You will likely prefer the Hawaii Diet eat-more approach or perhaps Jeff Novick's intuitive visuals. But no matter which approach you choose, the end is the same: being healthy, feeling full, and losing weight.

I was never hungry eating during the Rescue Week, and I still lost 8 pounds. Extremely amazed!
—James McVeigh, age 68, retired city treasurer,
North Ridgeville, Ohio

Understanding Volumetrics

The philosophy of eating more food while consuming fewer calories is demonstrated in the principle of Volumetrics, which was designed by a professor at Penn State University named Dr. Barbara Rolls. A triathlon friend explained to me that we typically eat the same weight in food every day, and that what's important is how filling the food is compared to its calorie content. He mentioned Barbara's book, *The Volumetrics Weight-Control Plan*, which I quickly devoured.

A number of studies in the book immediately struck me as vitally important. For example, in one, Dr. Rolls's colleagues at Penn State prepared an all-you-can-eat buffet for normal-weight women involving a variety of high- and low-energy-dense meals. For lunch on Monday, for instance, the women might have been given pasta salad with more noodles and fewer veggies (a high-calorie meal), while on Tuesday that pasta salad had fewer noodles and more veggies (a low-calorie meal). But no matter how the meals were prepared, the women all ended up eating the same weight of food—about 3 pounds a day. Nevertheless, on the lower-calorie days, the women felt just as satiated when compared to the higher-calorie days.

Volumetrics has a simple mission statement: We want to eat a healthy, nutritious diet while not constantly feeling hungry and obsessing about food. In more biological terms, we want to be able to eat a certain amount of food that activates the stretch receptors and density receptors in our stomachs, which let our brains know we're full and satiated.

Here's what people don't understand: feeling full has nothing to do with a food's caloric content and everything to do with a food's volume. I want to repeat that: feeling full has nothing to do with a food's caloric content and everything to do with a food's volume.

Let's do a quick science review. We hear the term "calories" all the time, but what does that word really mean? A calorie is a measure of the amount of heat produced when your digestive system metabolizes food. This heat produces the energy that powers your body. Caloric energy doesn't necessarily apply to just food. Anything that contains energy has calories. A ton of coal, for example, has the potential to burn more than 7 billion calories. Meanwhile, the total energy found in 770 cups of oatmeal could move a car 90 miles, and 18 tomatoes could power a lightbulb for 90 minutes.

Fortunately, humans require a lot fewer calories than electric power plants. But your body needs the energy found in food calories to survive; otherwise, your heart and other organs would stop working. As we'll see, a food's physical size has nothing to do with its caloric content. What matters is the food's components: One gram of carbohydrates has 4 calories; 1 gram of protein has 4 calories; and 1 gram of fat has 9 calories. Water, meanwhile, has 0 calories, and alcohol has 7 calories per gram.

Understanding Calories

When reading the nutrition facts label on a food, it's important to understand where the calories shown on the label are coming from. Remember: One gram of fat contains 9 calories, and 1 gram of carbohydrates and 1 gram of protein both have 4 calories. Let's take a look at a 348-calorie serving of eggs, which contains:

24 grams of fat, so 24 x 9 = 216 calories
31 grams of protein, so 31 x 4 = 124 calories
2 grams of carbohydrates, so 2 x 4 = 8 calories
Overall, 216 of your egg calories are coming from fat, 124 from protein, and 8 from carbs.
Now let's look at a 100-calorie apple:
0.3 grams of fat, so 0.3 x 9 = 2.7 calories
0.5 grams of protein, so 0.5 x 4 = 2 calories
24 grams of carbohydrates, so 24 x 4 = 96 calories

In this case, just over 2 calories are coming from fat, while 96 are coming from healthy unprocessed carbs.

The proportion of these components determines how calorie-dense a certain food is. The more fat, the more energy-dense; the more water, the less energy-dense.

Let's do a little thought experiment. Imagine taking a bowl and filling it with two cups of grapes. Then take another bowl and drop in just a quarter cup of raisins. Which would be more filling? The grapes, of course. You don't need a scale to know that the whole grapes weigh a lot more—and therefore fill you up better—than their dried counterparts. Nevertheless, those two cups of grapes and that quarter cup of raisins have the exact same amount of calories: 100. The nutrition might be the same, but you're feeling a whole lot more full when you choose the grapes (the whole food) instead of the raisins (the processed food).

Let's try another one. In the right corner, weighing in at a lean-and-mean 7 ounces, is a nice juicy whole tomato. In the left corner, a teensy 1-ounce serving of potato chips. You don't need to have seen all the *Rocky* flicks to know how this one ends. The 7-ounce tomato has just 32 calories, while the 1-ounce serving of chips has 152 calories. That's barely 14 percent of the tomato's weight, yet *475 percent* of the tomato's caloric content. What if we made this a fair fight and beefed up that serving of chips to equal the tomato's 7 ounces? Now you'd have to eat 33 large tomatoes to equal the same caloric hit. Any Little Leaguer can wolf down an 7-ounce bag of chips, but I'd pay to see even the baddest bodybuilder devour 33 whole tomatoes in one sitting.

Volumetrics asks you to do a little bit of math. Instead of calories, we're going to look at the number of calories in a given weight, in this case the *calories per gram*. This calculation allows you to circumvent deceptive food labels to determine how healthy your food is.

Don't worry. It's super easy. Just head to http://www.nutritiondata .com and look up the nutrition information of any food. Then divide the amount of calories per serving (the energy) by the grams per serving (the weight). For example, a serving of Mega Stuf Oreos has 180 calories and weighs 36 grams. So 180 divided by 36 gives you a calorie density of 5.0. Meanwhile, a watermelon has an energy density of 0.3 (one wedge contains approximately 87 calories and weighs 286 grams).

The lower the calorie density, the more likely the food is healthy. Ideally, we want to shoot for a calorie density under 1.5, where the vast majority of the strong food you'll be eating during the Seven-Day Rescue, such as fruits and vegetables, resides. Here are the calorie densities of some common foods:

Food	Calorie Density
Tomatoes	0.2
Broccoli	0.3
Carrots	0.4
Apples	0.5
Kale	0.5
Blueberries	0.6
Black beans	0.8
Sweet potatoes	0.8
Brown rice	1.1
Fried eggs	2.0
Beef	2.5

Food	Calorie Density
Swiss cheese	2.8
Plain M&Ms	4.9
Bacon	5.0
Butter	7.2
Olive oil	8.8

Eat More!

About ten years ago, I picked up an enlightening book called *The Hawaii Diet* by Terry Shintani (Terry took over the medical practice from plant-based superstar doctor John McDougall on the Big Island of Hawaii). For Dr. Shintani, health is more than just optimal cholesterol and blood pressure levels. *Happiness* levels are equally important. What good is being healthy if you're feeling miserable all the time? I see this with fad diets, where sitting down to eat often makes dieters depressed. You prepare pathetic, measly little meals that never fill you up, keeping you in a constant state of hunger. That's why the cover of Dr. Shintani's book states proudly: "Eat all you want." Hell yeah! Who doesn't love eating?

The crux of Dr. Shintani's program is this: no food deprivation. Eat as much as you want and still lose weight. Dr. Shintani's principles are actually quite similar to Volumetrics, although with less of an emphasis on math and food labels and more of an emphasis on spiritual, mental, and emotional happiness. And what better way to achieve happiness than by eating lots and lots of healthy plant food?

The Hawaii Diet introduced me to the Shintani Mass Index (SMI). Terry assigned every food a value based upon how many pounds of that food you would have to eat to consume 2,500 calories—roughly the amount most people eat in any given day—and maintain your current weight. I found it absolutely fascinating! For example, in order to maintain your weight just by eating carrots, you'd have to eat 13 pounds of them. In order to maintain your weight with eggplant, you'd have to eat about 29 pounds. But in order to get 2,500 calories from butter, you would have to eat just 0.8 pounds, or from chicken only 3 pounds!

Here are some more SMI values, the amount of each food eaten to get to 2,500 calories:

Weak Food	Strong Food
Bacon 0.8	Chick peas 5.6
Butter 0.8	Corn 6.5
Mayonnaise 0.8	Tofu 7.6
Almonds 0.9	Potatoes 9.6
Peanut butter 0.9	Collard greens 12.1
Cashews 1.0	Beets 12.7
Beef sirloin 1.2	Oranges 15.6
Donuts 1.3	Peaches 16.5
Eggs 1.3	Broccoli 17.1
Beef chuck 1.4	Cauliflower 20.2
Cheese (cheddar) 1.4	Asparagus 21.0
Danish pastry 1.5	Watermelon 21.0
Sugar 1.5	Cabbage 22.8
Ham sandwich 1.6	Artichokes 26.0
French fries 1.7	Tomatoes 27.3
Tuna (in oil) 1.9	Cucumbers 32.8
Pork 2.1	Lettuce 39.0

The key to losing weight *and* feeling fuller than ever before? Eat a wide variety of low-calorie-dense food. Imagine strutting into your local Weight Watchers meeting and informing the group that you ate 250 pounds of lettuce the previous week and *still* lost weight! That may sound silly, but it's against human evolution to willfully stop yourself from eating before you're full. As long as you choose strong, fibery, robust plant foods, you'll never have to worry about this conundrum again!

Here's a fun comparison. What do you think has more calories? A 14-ounce family-size bag of Lay's Classic Potato Chips or an enormous 9-pound watermelon?

Let's do the math. The chips have a whopping 2,100 calories, including an artery-busting 140 grams of fat and a heart-stopping 2,500 mg of sodium. All that destruction with just 14 ounces of food! Now let's check out the watermelon. Even though this bad boy weighs in at 9 pounds, it contains only 1,300 calories. Instead of 140 grams of fat, you're getting 7 grams. Instead of 2,500 mg of sodium, you're getting just 45 mg. Meanwhile, you're consuming 5,000 mg of potassium, 18 grams of fiber, 28 grams of protein, and nearly a week's worth of vitamins A and C. And I haven't even counted the nice workout you get from cutting that sucker into manageable portions! And which do you think will fill you up more?

I am a big guy (275 pounds) and I eat a lot. On Friday, through bad planning, I went from lunch at 1:00 p.m. until dinner at 10:00 p.m. and was amazed I was not starving! I was shocked driving home as I passed one fast-food place after another without even being tempted to stop. I was looking forward to a plant-strong dinner when I got home!
—Tom Kehoe, age 65, firefighter

How about scarfing down a whole cup of black beans? Assuming you could do it in one sitting, you'd rake in 2,760 mg of potassium, which is nearly 80 percent of your daily intake; 39 grams of protein, good for another 80 percent of your daily intake; and 29 grams of fiber, which is more than 115 percent of your daily intake! And for that massive injection of nutrition you're looking at just 624 calories—not bad! Compare that to a cup of peanut butter, which nets you 130 grams of fat, or 200 percent of your daily fat intake (including 135 percent of your saturated fat daily intake!); 24 grams of sugar; just 1,674 mg of potassium (47 percent of your daily intake); and just 15 grams of fiber. Oh, and you're also getting 1,518 calories in the process.

Remember, higher calories doesn't mean higher satiety. No matter the calorie content, you end up eating roughly the same volume of food every day. Indeed, studies in Europe and the United States have proved this. For example, an American survey asked participants to weigh their food every day for four days. Even though their choices of food varied substantially, the participants on average ate the same *weight* of food. A study of 7,356 adults published in the *American Journal of Clinical Nutrition* found that people eating a low-energy-dense diet—namely, one rich in fruits and vegetables—ate fewer calories per day (425 less for men, 275 less for women) compared to people eating a high-energy-dense diet. Another survey found that obese men and women tend to eat a lot of energy-dense food and scant amounts of energy-light food, and a Dutch study noted that its leanest participants had a much less energy-dense diet compared to obese participants.

In the meantime, people tend to have a terrible sense of how many calories they're eating. For instance, in a recent study published in the *BMJ*, researchers interviewed more than 1,800 adults and 1,100 teenagers in fast-food restaurants, asking them to estimate the caloric content of their meals. The study found that "at least two-thirds of all participants underestimated the calorie content of their meals, with about a quarter underestimating the calorie content by at least 500 calories." Adults on average underestimated the caloric content of their meals by 175 calories, and teenagers by 259.

So why exactly do low-energy-dense foods make us feel full despite not having lots of obesity-causing calories? It's a process that's as much psychological as it is physiological.

It begins with your eyes. If you head over to my house where I prepare for you a giant mound of brown rice smothered in black beans, sweet potato cubes, roasted corn, green onions, and topped with fresh salsa and avocado (Building Your Rescue Supper Bowl, page 233) and place it in front of you, your brain's going to say, "Oh, baby. This plate is *huge*. I'm going to feel so full afterward." The expectation of fullness can be just as important in filling you up as the actual meal is. Conversely, if you eat at a fancy all-raw restaurant where they slide you a $20 plate of nachos with six sprouted chips and a side of cashew sauce, you probably won't expect to feel very full afterward.

Next up, your eyes and mouth. When you get a whiff of that glorious rice dish—that mouthwatering mixture of black beans, sweet potatoes, roasted corn, green onions, salsa, and avocado—it's a sensory delight that's surpassed only by actually tasting the food. The more food on your plate, the longer you get to experience the pleasure of eating. But if that pleasure lasts for only a few moments, you're left wanting more.

And finally, the stomach. Inside it are stretch and density receptors, which are essentially a bunch of sensors that respond to the stretching of surrounding muscle tissue. The more food you eat, the more your stomach stretches and activates these sensors, which then tell your brain that you've eaten a satisfying amount of food. In the minutes and hours following a meal, your stomach contracts rhythmically, breaking down the food into tiny bits and pieces. The more food you consume, regardless of its calorie content, the longer it takes the stomach to break down the food and the longer you feel satiated. Then, as food moves through your small intestine, liver, pancreas, and other digestive organs, more satiety signals are sent to your brain. For instance, a satiety hormone is released by the small intestine when it encounters a large volume of food. The more food you eat, the longer you feel full.

In short, feeling full has nothing to do with the amount of energy in a food. In this particular case, size *does* matter.

So if not calories, what are low-energy-dense foods stuffed with to make them so hefty? Water. Remember that at 9 calories per gram, fat is the most energy-dense, while water has 0 calories. The more water bulking up your food, the heavier and more filling it will be. In chapter 1 we saw that many fruits and vegetables are more than 85 percent water, which means that at least 85 percent of their volume contains 0 calories. If you remember from earlier in this chapter, a quarter cup of raisins has the same 100 calories as two cups of grapes—that's a whopping eightfold difference in the quantity of food! The only difference is that the raisins are dried, while the grapes have retained their water.

If you're trying to lose weight, adding water-dense plant-strong food to your diet can work wonders. For example, in one study conducted by Penn State University, researchers took 101 obese women and divided them into two groups. Half decreased their fat intake while the other half decreased their fat intake and also increased their intake of water-rich fruits and veggies. After six months, the fruit-and-veggie group had lost more than 21 pounds on average despite consuming more food by weight than the reduced-fat-only group, who lost 15 pounds. What's more, the women in the fruit-and-veggie group reported feeling much less hungry and much more satiated overall. Guess which diet will be more sustainable?

In another study, this one published in *ISRN Obesity*, researchers found that through increasing fiber intake each day by the equivalent of 1.5 cups of beans, as well as increasing the intake of fruits and veggies, participants were able to decrease their caloric intake by 250 to 350 calories while "hunger was significantly reduced." Just by eating a whole-food, plant-based diet, you improve your health, lose excess weight, and feel full all the time. Sounds like a win-win-win situation to me!

Watermelon Bingeing

My friend Tim was a fellow firefighter with whom I had gone through the fire academy in 1997. Tim was one of the bigger cadets, weighing in at 235 pounds at the time—and after a decade in the fire department, he'd ballooned up to 304 pounds. Tim did what most firefighters do: gain between 5 and 10 pounds a year. This is easy to do when you're eating all the toxic foods abundant in the typical firehouse kitchen. To boot, most firefighters are still men, and the prevailing macho male mentality around food is protein, protein, protein, meat, meat, meat, fried, fried, fried, ice cream, ice cream, ice cream!

When I reached out to Tim to see if he would like to join my first pilot study back in 2008—in which participants ate only plant-strong food for twenty-eight days—he was excited. Tim hit it out of the park! And he was always super diligent about sending me his daily food log so I could make sure he was following the program 100 percent.

One day I noticed an odd entry. For dessert he wrote down "watermelon (the whole thing)." I sent Tim an e-mail asking if it was a small, personal-size watermelon and he wrote back, "No! A family-size watermelon!!"

Over the course of the twenty-eight days, Tim lost 33 pounds—more than any other participant. In addition, his cholesterol dropped down to 83 mg/dl and his LDL fell below 40 mg/dl. He achieved all of this while eating a staggering amount of strong, plant-based foods. Tim rocked it to the core. He understood what he could eat unlimited amounts of (watermelon!) and what he needed to steer clear of.

Eat like Tim, eat a lot like Tim, and get healthy like Tim!

A VISUAL APPROACH TO MAXIMIZING WEIGHT LOSS

One of the first times I heard the term "calorie density" was in 2010 when I started hosting Engine 2 Seven-Day Rescue Diet programs for Whole Foods Market employees. I had assembled an incredible team of doctors, psychologists, chefs, and personal trainers to help me educate participants about the ins and outs of eating strong food and living the plant-strong lifestyle. One of these experts was dietician/nutritionist Jeff Novick. Jeff was amazing at doing handstands (he consistently beat me at the end of the week when we had our annual handstand contest), but he was even more skilled at delivering extraordinarily educational and entertaining lectures. Much of this comes from his experience: Jeff has been teaching people the benefits of eating a whole-food, plant-based diet for more than thirty years! One of the most remarkable lectures in his arsenal is on calorie density. Jeff explains it in an easy-to-understand way that makes you feel like you can't wait to jump in, apply these principles to your plant-based life, and make them an ongoing habit.

Jeff's number one principle sums up why I respect him so much: "Whenever hungry, eat until you are comfortably full." Yes! No diet should starve you—I want you to eat, eat, eat until your stomach is full! You shouldn't have to wait until dinnertime to enjoy a healthy, delicious plant-strong meal.

We've used some math in the previous sections, but Jeff really gets to the point with a fantastic visual guide to filling your plate:

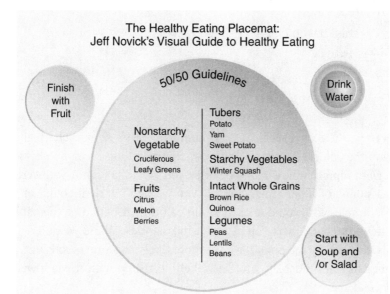

The Healthy Eating Placemat:
Jeff Novick's Visual Guide to Healthy Eating

50/50 Guidelines

Finish with Fruit

Drink Water

Nonstarchy Vegetable
Cruciferous
Leafy Greens

Fruits
Citrus
Melon
Berries

Tubers
Potato
Yam
Sweet Potato

Starchy Vegetables
Winter Squash

Intact Whole Grains
Brown Rice
Quinoa

Legumes
Peas
Lentils
Beans

Start with Soup and /or Salad

If you don't want math anywhere near your food, this approach is for you. Here it is from Jeff himself:

To find the sweet spot of calorie density at each meal, start with a soup and/or salad. Then make your plate (by visual volume) about 50 percent intact whole grains, roots/tubers, starchy vegetables, and beans. Make the other half nonstarchy vegetables and fruits. This gives you the perfect mix of low calorie density, high nutrient density, and high satiety.

The Calorie Density Scale

Foods	Calories per Pound
Vegetables	60–195
Fruit	140–420
Potatoes, pasta, rice, barley, yams, corn, hot cereals	320–630
Beans, peas, lentils (cooked)	520–780
Breads, bagels, fat-free muffins, dried fruit	920–1360
Sugars (e.g., sugar, honey, molasses, agave, corn syrup, etc.)	1200–1800
Dry cereals, baked chips, fat-free crackers, pretzels	1480–1760
Nuts/seeds	2400–3200
Oils	4000

If you are curious about the numbers, Jeff's simple chart above shows the calorie density of the most common foods. The numbers on the right represent how many calories you would take in if you were to eat 1 pound of a particular food. If you were to guzzle a pound of oil, for example, you would take in 4,000 calories. A pound of vegetables, on the other hand, nets you as few as 60 calories. While we don't typically eat food by the pound, we are more likely to overeat foods that are higher in calorie density and less likely to fill up with foods lower in calorie density.

As Jeff has pointed out, the balance of nutritional studies reveals that you can freely eat foods with a calorie density of 300 or less (vegetables, most fruits, and calorie-dilute meals under 300 calories per pound), and you can eat a significant amount of foods with a calorie density of 300 to 800, and not worry about gaining weight.

To make things even easier, Jeff has organized a list without any numbers at all:

Eat Freely:
(Foods Low in Calorie Density)
Fruits and veggies

Eat Relatively Large Portions without Concern:
(Foods Moderate in Calorie Density)
Starchy veggies, intact whole grains, and legumes

Limit These Foods:
(Foods High in Calorie Density)
Breads, bagels, dry cereals, crackers, tortillas, dried fruit

Extremely Limit These Foods:
(Foods Very High in Calorie Density)
Nuts, seeds, oils, solid fats, junk foods

When it comes to calorie-dense plant foods, Jeff recommends you think of them as condiments. You may add small amounts of avocado, walnuts, and raisins to your salad, for example, but they should never form the basis of any meal.

What About Nuts?

Most whole-plant foods are so calorie-dilute that you can eat as much as you want, whenever you want. With a few plant foods, however, you need to be careful.

For example, despite how delicious they may be, nuts are little fat bombs that have a horrific ratio of omega-6 fats to omega-3 fats—for example, almonds are 2,500 to 1—which can be a major contributor to heart disease–causing inflammation. For perspective, the ideal ratio of omega-6s to omega-3s is 1:1, 2:1, or 3:1. One of the reasons walnuts are our nut of choice is because they have a 3:1 ratio of omega-6s to omega-3s. Avocados are also overly high in fat, especially unhealthy fats: 15 percent saturated fat and 65 percent mono-unsaturated fat, while just the remaining 20 percent comes from essential polyunsaturated healthy fats.

When it comes to nuts, remember that they contain all the building blocks of a tree—fat, carbohydrates, and protein—all crammed into a tiny shell. (You wouldn't have many trees if nuts had the calorie density of tomatoes—you'd probably need seeds the size of cars!) Remember that with every nut, you're eating all the calories and nutrients needed to grow a tree!

This is the Engine 2 Diet: Eat whole foods. As much as you want. Only plants. As long as you follow the principles of calorie density outlined in this chapter, you'll never have to be hungry again while losing weight.

Eat more food and weigh less. This is what we all want. This is what is sustainable. This is what makes sense. This is the heart of the Engine 2 Seven-Day Rescue!

5

Why We Limit Protein

My great-grandfather George Washington Crile (1864–1943) is considered one of America's greatest doctors. He died long before I was born, but he still looms larger than life in my family. I remember bringing friends home after school and opening the *Encyclopaedia Britannica* (for all you millennials, that's how we got our information before the advent of Wikipedia) and showing him off. "The Chief," as he was called by his colleagues, was written about for many reasons but principally for performing the first successful blood transfusion from one human to another. He also cofounded the Cleveland Clinic in 1921, wrote all kinds of influential books, and invented several important medical techniques and tools. In World War II, the United States liberty ship SS *George Crile* was named in his honor.

In his two-volume autobiography, *George Crile*, my great-grandfather concluded the chapter titled "Hemorrhage and Transfusion" by mentioning how frustrated he was that thousands of lives could have been saved before and after World War I if the medical establishment had embraced his new procedure as a method of counteracting all forms of hemorrhage as well as depleted states—gravely injured soldiers simply couldn't produce enough blood to live without help from a transfusion. The sad reality is that it took more than three decades before transfusions became a commonplace practice by the medical establishment.

The chapter's last sentence hit me like a ton of cauliflower: "Such is the inertia of the human race." These eight words have stayed with me ever since. I particularly think about them when I hear of doctors prescribing an endless battery of dangerous prescription drugs for their cardiac patients instead of prescribing a whole-food, plant-strong diet—the only proven way to prevent, arrest, and reverse heart disease. I also think about my great-grandfather's words when I hear certain nutritional myths that have no grounding in science, such as that milk is good for your bones, or that you must eat oily fish to get enough omega-3 fatty acids. It's as if there's too much inertia out there for people to change their minds and accept the truth.

And the very worst myths of all involve protein. I get questions like these all the time:

"How do you get your protein with a plant-based diet? Only animal products have protein."

"Aren't plant-based proteins incomplete?"

"Don't you need lots of protein to build muscle?"

These assumptions are very wrong. During the question-and-answer session following a talk I gave in St. Paul, Minnesota, a teenager mentioned to me that he wanted to build more muscle mass. I asked him how he was structuring his workouts. He said he went to the gym three days a week and ate lots of protein daily to ensure he was building muscle. When I asked him what he was eating, he replied: bacon and eggs for breakfast; chicken breasts for lunch; and either steak, hamburger, or fish for dinner. To boot, he drank two muscle milk protein shakes during the day.

I could almost feel my arteries seizing up.

I asked him why in the world he had come to hear me talk with a diet like that and he replied that his mother had asked him to come.

I told him that not only was he overdosing on the wrong type of protein, but he was consuming far more protein than anyone needs. Moreover, it was *toxic* protein from animal sources, and nothing he was eating contained fiber, phytonutrients, carbohydrates, or antioxidants—all the things we need that are found in whole, plant-based foods. His meals were a weak cocktail of animal products and animal by-products, without any of the building blocks from plants that would allow him to flourish on the outside as well as the inside.

The kid was getting a firestorm of unhealthy animal protein, animal fat, and animal cholesterol in meal after meal. Bacon is nothing but fat and protein, and, much to the chagrin of the Paleo people—not to mention *Time* magazine, which proclaimed that "bacon is back"—it is not healthy. Meanwhile, eggs are not the perfect source of protein as many people have been led to believe. Eggs are a concentrated source of weak animal protein and cholesterol (one egg yolk has 212 mg/dl—the same as two Burger King Whoppers). In addition, close to 65 percent of an egg's calories come from fat, with over 20 percent coming from saturated fat. And I hate to break it to those of you who have been subsisting on skinless chicken breasts, but the leanest cuts are 30 percent saturated fat, have the same amount of cholesterol as red meat, and are riddled with weak and destructive animal protein. As my father likes to say, there is no such thing as lean meat, just less-fat meat.

And don't get me started on that muscle milk nonsense. This drink of choice for many bodybuilders is made mostly from bovine growth fluid (cow-milk proteins) mixed with a few extracted oils. I told that kid there was more than enough protein in every plant food to easily meet his needs. I informed him that consuming massive amounts of protein had nothing to do with getting big, ripped, and buff. Heck, if that were the case, all of America would be walking around looking like the Rock. And as we all know, more people are walking around looking like the Pillsbury Doughboy than Dwayne Johnson. After all, the average female takes in 70 grams of protein per day, and the average male takes in more than 100 grams! To put this in perspective, the Institute of Medicine, which advises the federal government, recommends that men consume 56 grams a day and women 46 grams.

Forget about the protein for a moment. The best way to get muscular and shredded is by taxing your muscles with either weight or resistance training, allowing recovery time, and then repeating this process so your muscles can adapt and grow according to the stresses placed on them. We've known this forever.

It also so happens that the crown jewels for muscle recovery and performance are whole-plant foods. Plants have healthy fats loaded with unprocessed carbohydrates (our dominant fuel source). Plants are brimming with micronutrients to defend against oxidative stress and inflammation. And plants rock the perfect amount of lean and healthy protein to keep your muscles strong. When I was a professional triathlete training between two and six hours a day for two decades, I never, ever worried about getting enough protein. Every time I was asked the question, "Where on earth do you get protein?," my answer was always the same: "BGP." Beautiful glorious plants. After the question-and-answer session I spoke with the boy and reassured him that, like many bodybuilders, UFC fighters, and NFL football players, he could get as big and strong as he wanted, without jeopardizing his health, with plant-strong foods as his muse. He broke into a wide grin and told me he was excited to get after it!

Let's move past our inertia, lose our unnatural cravings for animal flesh and animal secretions, and be done with it. Be done with pretending animal protein is the way to be strong. Be done with all the unnecessary and debilitating chronic diseases. It all starts with changing your fundamental perception on the issue of "Where will I get my protein if I don't eat meat or dairy products?"

Take a seat. Let's talk protein.

> Protein is available with a plant-based diet. Losing weight with the program was remarkably easy!
> —Jim Ziemnik, age 55, director of Lorain County, Ohio, metro parks

WHAT IS PROTEIN, ANYWAY?

Don't worry if this question popped into your head. If someone is going to tell you how much protein you need and where you should get your protein, it might help to know what protein actually is, right?

Protein is the body's building block, helping grow everything from bones and muscle to skin and hair. Protein makes up about 20 percent of your body weight—it's so plentiful that if you removed the water from your body, you'd be a whopping 75 percent protein. Protein itself is a molecule composed of much smaller building blocks called amino acids. These acids link themselves into chains to form individualized proteins with specific roles. Think of proteins like buildings, and amino acids like bricks. Each building serves a special purpose, and each building requires uniquely shaped and sized bricks arranged in a specific sequence.

Our bodies contain more than ten thousand different kinds of protein, each busy doing its own particular job. In addition to growing and repairing tissue, protein is necessary for the production of enzymes, hormones, and countless other body chemicals. Antibodies—blood proteins that counteract toxins and foreign substances in the body—support the immune system, and protein carriers aid in the transport of molecules, such as iron, in the blood.

To make proteins, the body needs amino acids—twenty of them, specifically. The good news is that we can synthesize eleven of them on our own, but the other eight—known as "essential" amino acids—must be taken in through our food. Every food on the planet has some protein, but the quality of the food depends on the amounts and ratio of the essential amino acids.

How much protein do we need? The official recommendation from the Institute of Medicine, a division of the National Academies of Sciences, Engineering, and Medicine, is 0.8 gram of protein per kilogram of body weight. So if you weigh 150 pounds, that comes out to 50 grams of protein per day, or 10 percent of your daily caloric intake. Nevertheless, most Americans get far more than they need. People eating the standard American diet often take in as much as 30 percent or more of their calories from animal protein, which, as you'll soon see, places an enormous burden on the bones, kidneys, and heart, and promotes cancerous tumors.

Plants, on the other hand, provide the ideal amount of protein without taxing your body's systems.

A Most Serious Obstacle in the History of Humanity

J. Morris Hicks, who wrote *Healthy Eating, Healthy World*, has this to say about our obsession with protein:

> Because of the mistaken, yet almost ubiquitous, belief that we humans actually "need" to eat animal protein to be healthy, incredibly powerful solutions to our sustainability crisis don't even make it to the table for consideration. For this reason, I consider that "protein myth" to be the most serious obstacle in the history of humanity. For if we cannot take the "animal out of the equation" when it comes to feeding humans...the future of our civilization (and even our species) is in peril.

THE PROTEIN MYTH

Peek your head into just about any fire station around the country and you'll discover that the "Real men eat meat" myth is alive and well. It's time once and for all to let people know that this is not just a myth, but a dangerous one that is burning down people's health.

I can't even begin to tell you how widespread the protein fallacy is. I have my Seven-Day Rescue participants fill out a survey before the program begins, and the most common concern is getting enough protein in their diet. One participant from the North Ridgeville, Ohio, study told me about how her athlete friends pontificate on the "quackery" of the plant-based lifestyle. They don't care that literally *every* food has protein, and that you can get all the protein you could possibly ever need from plants. They declare that you can get enough protein only by eating animal foods.

It's time to destroy this myth once and for all.

As mentioned, the typical American on the standard American diet may get as much as 30 percent of his or her calories from protein. The typical American is also among the least healthy in the world. Americans die at an earlier age than most Europeans and Japanese. We have much higher rates of obesity, heart disease, cancer, and diabetes. A 2013 report from the Institute of Medicine comparing US rates of death and disability to those of sixteen peer nations (including Canada, Australia, Japan, and the countries of Western Europe) found that Americans trail the rest of the developed world on virtually every measure of health and well-being. And, as of 2014, according to *U.S. News and World Report*, Americans have the distinction of being the fattest people on earth.

If you have time, check out the enlightening book *Proteinaholic* by Dr. Garth Davis, in which the author digs deep into the history of protein and why our country has grown to worship it at the altar. As Davis explains in his book, if you look at the Japanese island of Okinawa, you'll see residents consuming a high-unprocessed-carb, low-protein diet—in fact, just 7 percent of Okinawans' calories come from protein. Nevertheless, Okinawa enjoys the world's highest rates of centenarians and among the lowest rates of obesity. These people sip protein. We gorge it like it's coming out of a fire hose.

So how did this myth that we need piles of protein first emerge? Let's go back in time to find the answer. If you glance at any fashion magazine, you'll see today's bodies held to an impossibly chiseled standard—men with perfect six-packs and ripped pecs, women with impeccably toned thighs and Barbie-doll waists. But if you look throughout history, you'll find the opposite was once true. Being heavy used to be a sign of wealth. The bigger your gut, the bigger your wallet! In most cultures, meat was considered a luxury, and the more you ate, the richer (and the fatter) you must be. Nowadays people poke fun at presidential candidates who tip the scales, but obese presidents like Grover Cleveland and William H. Taft were once admired for their prosperity and power. Even the word *protein* itself reflects self-worth—it comes from the Greek word *proteos*, meaning "of prime importance."

It also didn't help that when the nutrient protein was first isolated in 1839 by Dutch chemist Gerhard Mulder, it was taken from meat. This led to the erroneous belief that *only* meat had this nutrient of "prime importance." Later, the renowned German physiologist Carl von Voit declared that adult men needed an absurd 118 grams of protein per day, even though privately von Voit admitted this figure should be more like 52 grams per day. But von Voit's recommendation was influential, and to this day protein has been inextricably linked to meat, and lots of it—and both protein and meat have been equally inextricably linked to a false sense of good health.

As T. Colin Campbell points out, in the late 1800s researchers discovered that plants also contained protein, but the so-called experts dismissed these as "low-quality" sources. Why? In a society that associated body fat with prosperity, animal-based proteins were found to add fat at a faster pace than plant-based proteins. This finding was actually 100 percent accurate. But as we now know, excess body fat is a precursor to most chronic diseases.

Throughout the twentieth century, researchers poked holes in the protein myth. One of the first to do so was Russell Chittenden, a chemist at Yale University. Using a host of clinical trials (or, as we sometimes call it, *actual science*), Chittenden proved that young men who ate a low-protein, mostly plant-based diet were more physically conditioned compared to young men on a high-protein, animal-based diet.

The medical establishment just laughed at Chittenden, much the way they laughed at my great-grandfather's blood transfusion idea, but I know a few people who didn't get the memo that you need to gorge yourself with protein to be a top athlete. Just ask Rich Roll, who has twice finished near the top of the Ultraman World Championships, an insanely grueling, three-day triathlon featuring a 6.2-mile ocean swim, a 270-mile bike ride, and a 52.4-mile run. Ask the former British heavyweight boxing champion of the world, David Haye. Ask German strongman Patrik Baboumian, who broke the world record for most weight carried by a human being when he heaved 1,200 pounds across a 10-meter stage. Ask Alexey Voevoda, the Russian-born 250-pound double gold medalist in the bobsled at the Sochi 2014 Winter Olympic Games, who is also an eleven-time world arm-wrestling champion. Or how about MMA fighters Mac Danzig, Jake Shields, and James "Lightning" Wilks? I don't think my good friend Scott Jurek, the renowned ultramarathoner who recently broke the record for the fastest Appalachian Trail thru-hike (or should I say *run*: 2,160 miles in 46 days, 8 hours, 7 minutes), got the memo either. The sports might be different, but the results are the same: elite-level athletic performance on a 100 percent plant-strong diet.

Our Paradoxical Obsession with Protein

In his book *Proteinaholic*, Dr. Garth Davis, an expert surgeon specializing in weight loss, perfectly sums up our paradoxical obsession with protein:

Protein is everywhere. Big deal. So what is the problem? In a word: confusion. Some of us eat protein to lose weight, while others eat protein to gain weight. Ponder that paradox for a second. The same product sold to people to lose weight is relabeled and sold to others to gain weight! There are many who believe eating protein will make them healthier and help them live longer. And everybody seems to think protein will give them energy. Meanwhile, anyone who knows the basics of biochemistry or physiology will tell you that energy comes from carbs or fat, not protein. Possibly even more frightening is the fact that protein is one of the few food items that everyone seems to agree on. "Experts" argue about good fats and bad fats, or good carbs and bad carbs. This is very much part of the reason we are so confused about what to eat. But in protein we all seem to feel safe. No one would dare to argue that protein is bad for you.

Let's bust another myth right now, the one that claims people on plant-based diets don't get enough protein. Once again, we'll consult the actual science instead of folktales—or "bro science," as my buddy *Ultimate Fighter* winner James Wilks likes to say. The *Journal of the Academy of Nutrition and Dietetics* recently published results from the largest-ever study of people eating plant-based diets, comparing the nutrient profiles of 30,000 meat eaters and 25,000 individuals with predominantly plant-based diets. The meat eaters, of course, shoveled down protein by the truckload, but even people on strictly plant-based diets took in 70 percent more protein per day than is actually required. In other words, you can get all the protein you need just by eating plants.

Meanwhile, a panel that included the Food and Agriculture Organization and the World Health Organization concluded that "all usual food proteins would readily meet and even exceed the requirement for indispensable amino acids." In short, almost *any* diet will provide you essential amounts of protein. But, as we'll see later, only one diet provides you with *healthy* amounts of protein.

Pop quiz: Which has more protein per calorie, beef or broccoli? Yup. Broccoli. This green bodybuilding machine has 15.5 percent more protein per calorie than beef. But that doesn't stop your protein-seeking brainwashed neighbor from eating pounds of steak at a time.

Let's take a gander at the amount of protein in a few of the basic plant-based food groups, starting with leafy greens. Believe it or not, kale, broccoli, bok choy, and other cruciferous greens hover close to 35 percent protein, and spinach clocks in at a jaw-dropping 51 percent protein. Your average unassuming white mushrooms don't like to brag, but they're 57 percent protein. Your average intact whole grains, such as wheat, barley, millet, and rye, are 15 percent protein, with the ancient Peruvian grain quinoa setting the bar at 18 percent protein. Your typical legumes—black beans, split peas, red lentils, and pinto beans—are 25 percent protein, with soybeans taking the cake at over 40 percent. Your average fruit is 6 percent protein, though lemons steal the show at 16 percent.

When life gives you lemons, you get protein!

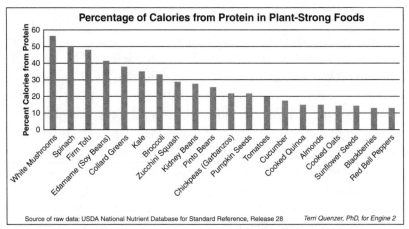

For those of you who think there's no protein in mushrooms or other plants, I say you're full of shitake! (For a more comprehensive protein chart, refer to Appendix 4.)

Now that you know the numbers, I want you to know that none of it really matters. Oops! This is because only 5 to 10 percent of our calories should come from protein. The higher end of that range is for pregnant women, who are giving some of their protein to another human, and athletes, who are actively breaking down and then having to build muscle. Nevertheless, as you can see from the list above, it would be virtually impossible for you to get less than 10 percent of your calories from protein. Any combination of fruits, vegetables, green leafy vegetables, beans, and whole grains will do!

Furthermore, when you're eating plants, you're also consuming all their other beneficial ingredients, such as fiber, vitamins, minerals, antioxidants, and phytonutrients. These are the superheroes you want coursing through your body when it comes to fighting off oxidative stress, building healthy cells, strengthening your immune system, and reversing disease.

Here's the simple truth: Plants have protein, they have plenty of it, and it's 100 percent healthy. Since you have a choice, why not choose the healthiest option? As Dr. Walter Willett, chair of Harvard's Department of Nutrition, recommends: "Pick the best protein packages by emphasizing plant sources of protein rather than animal sources."

Getting Enough Protein As an Athlete

If you exercise often, does that mean you need to take in more protein than if you don't? The answer is yes, but you don't have to go out of your way to find it. In fact, when you work out you generally increase your appetite and end up eating more food—and, therefore, you are eating more protein.

Because I'm quite physically active, instead of eating the typical 2,000 calories a day and consuming 50 grams of protein, I consume 3,000 calories and 75 grams of protein. Let me illustrate how easy this is to do just by increasing a few things you might eat during the day. If you boost the size of your morning oatmeal by half a cup and add in a small handful of walnuts, that will give you an extra 12 grams of protein. If you have one extra piece of whole-grain toast with hummus and veggies on top, that will give you an extra 11 grams of protein. If you have an extra 2 ounces of whole-grain pasta with your pasta primavera, you get an extra 7 grams of protein. If you decide to eat an extra 2 ounces of the latest bean or lentil pastas on the grocery store shelves, you'll take in an extra 18 grams of protein.

Just add a little more food at breakfast, lunch, and dinner, and you've got another 30 to 42 grams of protein. Don't change the food. Just change the portions.

Unless you're stuck on a desert island or otherwise trying to starve yourself, it's just about impossible to eat a protein-deficient diet. Protein deficiency is so rare that almost no one has ever even heard the word for it (kwashiorkor).

And yet I still have firefighter friends who are convinced that if they don't consume their daily ration of ham and eggs, tuna fish, chicken breast, steak, hamburger, cheese, and roast beef, they'll get weak and have to be hospitalized for protein deficiency.

Baloney!

The truth is, these are the exact foods that are responsible for an overmedicated America, an obese America, a sick America, a bankrupt America, a depressed America, and a dying America. Animal protein does not just provide your body with unnecessary protein, it provides it with *dangerous* protein. Here's why:

ANIMAL PROTEIN IS BAD TO THE BONE

We already destroyed the milk-is-good-for-you myth back in chapter 3. Want more? A study published in the *BMJ* followed about 100,000 people for two decades and concluded that drinking lots of milk, which is chock-full of animal protein at 8 grams per cup, was associated with a much higher risk of bone and hip fractures, not to mention up to twice the risk of death, more heart disease, and more cancer.

The problem lies with acid. Just like a swimming pool, your body's natural pH level can rise and fall. As your fluids become too acidic, your body is forced to compensate by extracting minerals from bones and tissue to bring down the acid level. Any guess which mineral is your body's first line of defense? It's calcium. Remember, calcium is an essential mineral that promotes healthy bones. Your body does not make it, so it must come from diet.

Calcium is also a fantastic antacid. If you've ever suffered from acid reflux, you probably took an over-the-counter medication like Tums or Rolaids, also known as...calcium carbonate. By swallowing calcium pills, you're making your body less acidic. Of course, you have your own internal supply of these pills in your bones. This means that every time your body gets a little too acidic, calcium is slowly leaching out of your skeleton to solve the problem. And if your body is always acidic, your bones can become brittle.

So what causes the body to become acidic? You guessed it: animal protein! We've actually known for a century that meat is acid-forming, and experiments as far back as the 1920s have demonstrated that eating meat causes a big spike in calcium in urine. It didn't get there by chance—that calcium is leached directly from your bones to heal your body every time you eat animal food. Indeed, a Harvard University study published in the *American Journal of Epidemiology*, which followed more than 80,000 women for twelve years, noted that animal protein was directly associated with an increased risk of forearm fracture, though this risk was not present for plant protein.

Meat, fish, dairy, poultry, and eggs almost universally have high levels of sulfur-containing amino acids, which are metabolized by the body into sulfuric acid. The more sulfuric acid in the body, the more calcium your body needs to neutralize it. Based on twenty-six similar studies, for every 40 grams of protein added to your diet, you pee out 50 mg of calcium. Considering your skeleton holds only about 2 pounds of calcium, over the course of a lifetime your frame grows weaker and weaker. Based on that math, people who wolf down 100 grams of protein per day could pee out most of the calcium in their bones within twenty-five years.

For strong bones, don't pay attention to those "Got milk?" ads, or anything else the dairy industry has to say. Plant-strong means bone-strong!

Getting Calcium from Plants

Remember, it's not called "cow-cium." It's called *calcium*. Since we can't make it on our own, we need to get it from diet. But contrary to what the dairy industry would like you to think, you can take in more than enough calcium from plants. Indeed, the Harvard Nurses' Health Study, one of the largest and longest-running investigations of factors that influence women's health, concluded that "fracture rates were higher for those who consumed three or more servings [of milk], compared to those who did not drink milk."

As T. Colin Campbell discovered in his China Study, even though rural Chinese consume practically no dairy products—and as a result take in about half the calcium compared to Americans—osteoporosis among these populations is practically nonexistent. That's because plant eaters get all the calcium they need from plant sources. And not only do plants offer plenty of calcium, they offer *better* calcium: the calcium in plants is absorbed twice as well as the calcium from milk.

To maximize your healthy sources of calcium, eat lots of green leafies, especially boiled collards (266 mg of calcium per cup) and kale (101 mg of calcium per cup), and legumes such as navy beans (127 mg of calcium per cup), white beans (161 mg of calcium per cup), and great northern beans (120 mg of calcium per cup). Fortified soy milk, meanwhile, offers 368 mg of calcium per cup, and 4 ounces of tofu (raw, firm) can deliver up to 750 mg of calcium, depending on how it is prepared.

The recommended daily intake of calcium is 1,000 mg, which is no problem at all with so many plant options available. Repeat with me again: plant-strong means bone-strong!

ANIMAL PROTEIN IS BAD FOR YOUR KIDNEYS

The kidneys might be the most underappreciated organs in the human body. They're working 24 hours a day, 365 days a year to perform an unsexy but critical task: filtering your blood and creating urine. Without our little bean-shaped buddies, waste products will accumulate in our blood and eventually kill us. Though they are small—each kidney is about the size of your fist—these mighty organs filter 150 quarts of blood every single day, nonstop.

If taken care of properly, your kidneys should last a lifetime. After all, you have two of them. Heck, if you're a real stand-up guy or gal, you can give one away to someone in need and still live a completely normal life. Sadly, though, most Americans don't take care of their kidneys: A recent survey published in *JAMA* found that only 41 percent of Americans tested had healthy kidney function. By age sixty-five, one in three Americans can expect to be suffering from chronic kidney disease. Eventually, kidneys can fail entirely, which means several times a week you have to undergo a laborious procedure called dialysis, during which a machine artificially filters your blood. It's inconvenient and not especially effective: the average life expectancy for someone on dialysis is less than three years.

There is no reason you should ever have to resort to dialysis. Like heart disease, diabetes, and so many other chronic diseases, kidney failure can be seen as a choice—a choice that comes down to what you put on your plate. Think of your kidneys as a car engine. If you take care of your engine, change the oil regularly, and don't drive too harshly, you can expect it to have a nice, long, trouble-free life. But if you treat your car like you're racing the Daytona 500 and constantly rev your engine past the red line, it won't last long.

Eating animal products inundates your kidneys with animal protein, causing massive inflammation and pushing the kidneys into a frenzied state called hyperfiltration as they go into overdrive to sift out the bad from the good. Our kidneys evolved to enter hyperfiltration once in a great while—after a rare hunt, perhaps—but they were never meant to continuously handle an unrelenting load of animal protein.

For example, a study published in the leading nephrology journal *Nephrology Dialysis Transplantation* concluded that beef, chicken, and fish cause the kidneys to enter hyperfiltration. On the other hand, plant-based protein does not. A recent study by Japanese researchers found that tuna fish causes kidney filtration rates to skyrocket by up to 36 percent within three hours of consumption. However, the equivalent amount of protein from tofu does not cause any noticeable strain on kidney function. It's no wonder that a review published in the *Clinical Journal of the American Society of Nephrology* of a study comprising thousands of participants concluded that kidney decline was directly associated with eating lots of animal protein, while no such decline was associated with plant protein.

What I love most of all about plants is that they not only prevent chronic disease, they can actively halt it. This is true for heart disease, and it can be true for kidney disease as well. Even if your kidneys have been revving up past that hyperfiltration red line for years, you can ease their burden right now by cutting animal protein out of your diet. So far, six clinical trials have proved that replacing animal protein with plant protein can immediately reduce hyperfiltration, and a 2014 double-blind, randomized, placebo-controlled trial published in *Clinical Biochemistry* proved that plant protein can help revive failing kidneys.

So why not do your bean-shaped buddies a favor and cut out the meat? They deserve it!

Preventing Kidney Stones

Anyone who has grown up on the standard American diet might have at some point in his or her life experienced kidney stones—those crystallized, pebble-size deposits that form in kidneys and can block the flow of urine. Kidney stones can be extremely painful and, if they grow too large, may need to be surgically removed.

Not that long ago kidney stones were rare, but today they are common: Since World War II, we've seen a massive increase in kidney stone cases coinciding with an equally massive increase in animal protein consumption.

Proving this link in a trial published in the journal *Clinical Science*, researchers had participants consume extra animal protein each day—the equivalent of about a can of tuna fish—and within two days the levels of kidney stone–forming compounds skyrocketed, boosting their kidney stone risk by 250 percent. Meanwhile, a 2014 Oxford University study found that plant eaters "have a lower risk of developing kidney stones compared with those who eat a high meat diet."

Lots of plants means no stones to pass.

ANIMAL PROTEIN AND CANCER

I'll bet you thought the effects of animal protein on your bones and kidney were bad enough. But animal protein also acts as rocket fuel for cancer.

There are approximately 37 trillion cells in your body, and every single day your body creates 50 billion new ones and wipes out 50 billion old ones. It sounds incredibly violent, but it's just biology.

Children's bodies pump out more cells than they discard since they need extra cells to grow organs and limbs. But as adults, we don't want any excess cells wandering around the body, since they'll find their way to tumors who thirst for growth.

The body signals cells to grow, baby, grow, with a hormone called IGF-1. As kids, we have lots of IGF-1 running around to encourage cell division, but as adults our bodies dial back the IGF-1 so that we don't create more cells than we kill off. However, the body can also trigger the release of IGF-1 when it comes into contact with...drumroll...animal protein! When you consume it, animal protein stimulates IGF-1 production, your body pumps out more cells than it needs, and these extra cells then fuel the one thing left growing in your body: tumors.

IGF-1 is especially associated with prostate cancer. A meta-analysis of forty-two studies published in the *International Journal of Cancer* concluded that "raised circulating IGF-1 is positively associated with prostate cancer risk." And before any meatheads try to claim that both animal and plant proteins stimulate IGF-1, take a gander at this study published in the prestigious journal *Cancer Epidemiology, Biomarkers & Prevention*: After studying both meat eaters and plant eaters, the researchers concluded that animal protein was "positively associated with serum IGF-1," while a "plant-based diet is associated with lower circulating levels of total IGF-1." Animal protein increases your cancer risk while plant protein decreases it. It's as simple as that.

But remember, plant-strong means you have to be truly strong. You can't be kinda, sorta, sometimes strong. The more plant-strong you are, the more you reap the anticancer benefits of plants. Animal protein is in every animal food, no matter if it's meat, chicken, fish, milk, or egg whites. Within just two weeks of going cold turkey on not just turkey but all animal food, you can expect your IGF-1 levels to drop by as much as 20 percent. But the science shows that your occasional, willy-nilly, sometimes-maybe, Monday-Wednesday-Friday plant eaters are not able to meaningfully drop their IGF-1 levels.

Remember, folks: Go for all plants. All seven days. Yes. You. Can! Eat strong protein from plants!

Animal Protein and Heart Disease

A Harvard University study published a few years ago cut right to the meat of the matter: "Dietary protein and risk of ischemic heart disease in middle-aged men." After studying more than 43,000 men, what was the verdict?

It's right there on the first page: "Higher intake of animal protein may be associated with an increased risk of [ischemic heart disease] in 'healthy' men." Moreover, the researchers "observed a significant inverse association between higher vegetable protein intake and risk of fatal heart disease." In other words: more animal food, more heart disease; more plants, less heart disease.

This charade surrounding animal-based proteins is as intense as a Labrador retriever puppy playing fetch. Every day people are doubling up on chicken breasts, chugalugging protein powders, spooning down Greek yogurts, and gobbling up protein bars, convinced they are doing themselves and their bodies a favor.

We have this perverted notion that there is no such thing as enough protein. This isn't surprising. Everywhere we turn, we are bombarded with commercials and information touting the benefits of protein, even protein-enhanced shampoo and protein-infused baby food. During the 2014 Super Bowl, we watched the Rock dive through a plate-glass window and declare that we need to drink milk for protein.

Enough is enough. People should know the real story. We've been bombarded with so much pro-protein propaganda for so many decades that trying to convince anyone we don't need meat or dairy is like saying the sky is green and the grass is blue. It's tough for people to wrap their brains around this concept because it's a 180-degree difference from the prevailing cultural messages. We need some serious deprogramming.

I challenge you to surrender everything you think you know about nutrition, especially when it comes to the best, safest, and strongest sources of protein. We have to break free from this notion that the more protein we consume, the better. It isn't better. "More protein" is responsible for more chronic Western disease than any one of us can imagine.

Don't play the protein game any longer. Just say NO to animal protein as you would to crack, meth, or heroin. This is your brain on drugs, and these are your bones, kidneys, heart, and tumors on meat. Too many people in this country are animal protein junkies. It's time for America to visit a new "dealer" for our protein needs. His street name is Bro Broccoli. He or she also goes by other pseudonyms, such as King Quinoa, Queen Kale, Warrior of Watermelons, Duke of Dates, and the Princess of Peaches. Remember, you are getting all the junk that's keeping you down and messed up when you consume animal flesh, whether it's red meat, chicken, fish, pork, or eggs.

When it comes to animal protein, just say no!

Are Plant Proteins Complete?

Another crazy myth out there is that plant protein is somehow inferior to animal protein. Why? Well, people say it's because plant protein is not "complete." The argument goes that plant protein doesn't contain all of the essential amino acids that we need to be healthy, and that we have to eat a very specific combination of plants—or add in animal meat—to get our "complete" share of protein.

This is entirely, 100 percent untrue, but this myth is rampant not just on the Internet, but even in many medical textbooks and nutrition classes that still maintain plant protein is inferior to animal protein. Way back in the early 1900s experiments on rats (which require an entirely different set of nutritional requirements) formed the basis of this belief, and it was fueled by the popular 1971 book *Diet for a Small Planet* by Frances Moore Lappé. The author was neither a doctor nor a nutritionist. She was a sociologist aiming to eradicate world hunger. Although she had the best intentions, Lappé inadvertently promoted the myth that plant eaters need to eat a large, complex portfolio of plants every day in order to stay healthy.

Ten years later, when confronted with the truth about plant proteins, Lappé retracted this claim. But the belief has stubbornly persisted even in prestigious medical journals. For instance, in the journal *Circulation*, the Nutrition Committee of the American Heart Association erroneously declared that "although plant proteins form a large part of the human diet, most are deficient in one or more essential amino acids and are therefore regarded as incomplete proteins."

It's time to put this dangerous fallacy to bed once and for all. As the American Dietetic Association says, "Plant sources of protein alone can provide adequate amounts of the essential and nonessential amino acids." My friend Jeff Novick has also thoroughly debunked the claim that plant proteins are not complete. He writes: "You will find that any single whole natural plant food, or any combination of them, if eaten as one's sole source of calories for a day, would provide all of the essential amino acids and not just the minimum requirements but far more than the recommended requirements."

Once you move past your inertia, you'll discover plant protein is complete, it's completely perfect, and it's completely healthy.

6

Why We Limit Salt, Sugar, and Fat

Salt, sugar, fat. All three are essential to our health. All three can also be thoroughly destructive to our health. The difference lies in the amount we take in. A little bit of each is healthy, but Americans are overdosing on them like it's our job. Every day we shovel truckloads of the stuff into our bellies, often without even realizing it.

Why? Because food companies inundate even the most innocent-looking products, including staples like bread, with appetite-stimulating salt, sugar, and fat to make us addicted—so we buy more, and still more, and even more.

Most Americans don't have a clue that they're being led around grocery stores with a ring in their noses and a sign on their foreheads that screams "Sucker!" We haven't learned how to outwit, outsmart, and outplay the food companies at their own game. When you play by their rules, you become victim to the megadoses of salt, sugar, and fat these companies add to their products to make them taste better, to extend shelf life, and to get you hooked on their products.

Think I'm joking? Take a look at the best-selling book *The End of Overeating* by Dr. David Kessler, FDA commissioner under Presidents Clinton and Bush. In his book, Dr. Kessler describes in gory detail how food companies put salt on top of sugar on top of fat and then put more salt, sugar, and fat on top of the existing salt, sugar, and fat, all to get you addicted to their food—just as an alcoholic becomes addicted to alcohol or a heroin addict becomes addicted to heroin.

Likewise, read Pulitzer Prize–winning author Michael Moss's book *Salt Sugar Fat*, in which he describes how the "food giants have hooked us; hook, line and sinker." The stakes are high and these companies are playing for keeps. Their concern is their bottom line. They have little concern if you flatline.

But, you ask, what's the big deal? After all, salt, sugar, and fat make food taste great, right? They make everything sweet and juicy and sumptuous and...

Stop right there!

My goal during the Seven-Day Rescue is to throw you off your salt, sugar, and fat habit. Your eyes will open and your palate will awaken to the glorious and sublime flavors that naturally exist in whole, strong, plant-based foods. This means I am going to show you everything you need to know about how salt, sugar, and fat wreck your diets, your taste buds, and your health.

SALT

Table salt. An American tradition. What home in America doesn't have a salt shaker on the dinner table? Surely it can't be bad for us. It's not even an animal product. Salt, or sodium chloride, is a chemical compound containing a metal (sodium) and a halogen (chlorine). By weight, 3.5 percent of our planet's oceans are pure salt. How bad can it be? Well, according to a 2012 review in the *Lancet*, consuming too much salt may be killing up to 9 million people worldwide every year. That's roughly the population of Sweden.

The Institute of Medicine and the American Heart Association recommend that people not consume more than 1,500 mg of sodium a day. To put that in perspective, 1 teaspoon of salt is 2,300 mg of sodium. Believe it or not, most people are inhaling between *3,500* and *5,000* mg of sodium each and every day.

Of course the food industry can't get enough of salt. As Michael Moss points out in *Salt Sugar Fat*, Cargill, the number one supplier of salt, boasts in its sales literature that "people love salt. Among the basic tastes—sweet, sour, bitter, and salty—salt is one of the hardest ones to live without. And it's no wonder. Salt helps give foods their taste appeal—in everything from bacon, pizza, cheese and French fries to pickles, salad dressing, snack foods and baked goods."

So, yes, salt is great... for selling food. Not for selling health. Notice that the Cargill folks loved touting the sales benefits of salt, yet they fail to mention any *health* benefits from dumping mountains of addictive salt into food products. That's because there aren't any benefits to eating that much salt! Now, a bit of sodium is essential to optimal human health: Among many other benefits, sodium helps to maintain electrical currents among our muscles and nerves, regulate blood pressure, and sustain a healthy blood pH level. But in this case, too much of a good thing spells Trouble with a capital *T.*

Let's put our sodium consumption in historical context. We wolf it down now, but for 90 percent of human evolution our diets contained the equivalent of about a quarter-teaspoon of salt per day. That's because we ate plants, which contain only trace amounts of sodium. It wasn't until we learned how to preserve unhealthy animal meat using unhealthy amounts of salt that our sodium consumption really skyrocketed.

So if our bodies are meant to consume ten times less sodium than we consume now, what kind of bad stuff is going on under the hood?

Ingesting less sodium takes a lot of pressure off your body—blood pressure, that is. When you get your blood pressure taken at the doctor's office, you'll get two numbers back. Let's take mine, for instance, which is around 116/66 mm/Hg. The first number is my systolic blood pressure, meaning the pressure in my arteries when my heart is actively pumping blood. The second number, diastolic blood pressure, is the pressure in my arteries when my heart is resting between beats. Ideally, according to the American Heart Association, we should have a blood pressure below 120/80. Someone is considered to have high blood pressure if his or her reading is more than 140/90.

> My husband and I added more non-salt seasoning in one week than we have in a year. We made "French fries" with no oil and no salt and they were delicious!
> —Jackie Plantner, age 38, high school principal

High blood pressure, also called hypertension, is known as a "silent killer" because in most cases it has no symptoms. People with elevated blood pressure are straining their hearts by making them work harder to move blood around. Their hearts sweat and pound and gasp away, but they're none the wiser. For this reason, the Global Burden of Disease Study, which involved more than 300 institutions in 50 countries, concluded that high blood pressure is the number one worldwide risk factor for death, resulting in fatal heart attacks, strokes, and other catastrophic organ failures.

The basic problem with salt is that it encourages fluid retention in the body. Normally, your kidneys deploy a precise balance of potassium and sodium to remove extra water from the blood. But when you consume too much salt, this fragile sodium–potassium balance is shot to smithereens. As a result, your kidneys remove less water from your system. This puts damaging pressure on blood vessels in your kidneys, and your arteries bulge to accommodate the extra fluid. Tiny muscles in your arteries beef up in an attempt to support the extra pressure, but this only makes the blood passageways smaller—which both increases blood pressure and contributes to plaque buildup. Like a water main bursting under too much pressure, your arteries can burst suddenly without warning.

There are all sorts of little white pills out there that supposedly reduce your blood pressure, but you can reduce it much further, and much better, by cutting out those little white rocks—salt. An analysis in the *BMJ* calculated that if we could reduce our salt intake by a measly ½ teaspoon per day, we could prevent 22 percent of fatal strokes and 16 percent of fatal heart attacks. And when a study in the *New England Journal of Medicine* proclaims that "a reduction in salt intake of 3 [grams] per day"—that's a little bit less than 1 teaspoon—"would save 194,000 to 392,000 quality-adjusted life-years and $10 billion to $24 billion in health care costs annually," we should probably listen.

The evidence is clear. Don't let any salt sellers tell you otherwise! For example, the *Lancet* published a double-blind, randomized trial— the gold standard of clinical research—proving that if you ask people with high blood pressure to cut out their sodium, their blood pressure plummets. But if you give them *more* sodium, their blood pressure skyrockets. A study published in *Kidney International* demonstrated how just a single salty meal can massively increase blood pressure. The subjects were given a bowl of soup with a typical amount of salt, and within three hours their blood pressures surged. The folks who got soup with no added salt, however, did not suffer any such spike. And this is not new news: Way back in the 1940s, Duke University's famed diet researcher Dr. Walter Kempner was able to bring patients with horrendous blood pressures—as high as 240/150—down to 105/80 just by shifting them to a rice-and-fruit diet.

Is High Blood Pressure Normal?

I don't want to hear any baloney about high blood pressure being "normal," "genetic," or (boy, do I hate this one) "age-related." If your doctor says it's normal for blood pressure to increase with age and that this increase has nothing to do with diet, then get a new doctor! High blood pressure is *not* normal. Go to www .plantbaseddoctors.org and look up the nearest lifestyle doctor in your neck of the woods.

If you take your trusty sphygmomanometer over to the Amazon rain forest and spend some time hanging out with the Yanomami Indians, you'll find that their blood pressures *never* creep over 100/60. In an investigation known as the Intersalt Study, researchers could not find a single case of high blood pressure among this population of more than 10,000 men and women ages twenty to fifty-nine. *Not a single case.*

Why? Because Yanomami Indians get their sodium from only whole-plant foods. There are no Cheetos plants or Pringles roots in the rain forest. Just good old fruits and vegetables.

The science is clear: Too much sodium leads to high blood pressure, which leads to an early death. So, cut out the table salt. That's that, right?

Well, it's not that easy. Back in 1991, a groundbreaking study in the *Journal of the American College of Nutrition* revealed that saltshakers supply only about 6 percent of our overall sodium intake. Instead, the biggest source of sodium is right at the grocery store. The study found that a whopping *75 percent* of Americans' sodium comes from processed foods like mac and cheese, canned soups, salad dressings, tomato sauce, and pizza.

One surprisingly large contributor to America's sodium intake is humble bread. Here's a fun fact for you: Did you know that there is more sodium in one measly slice of Wonder Whole Grain White Bread (150 mg) than in one eighteen-chip serving of Lay's Oven Baked Potato Crisps (135 mg)? In fact, bread can contain as much as three times more sodium than potato chips.

How can this be? You can taste the salt from chips marinating on your tongue's ten thousand taste buds—that's what makes chips so deliciously addictive—but who's ever tasted the salt in bread? You don't, and that's the whole point. The salt in bread is baked into the flour and yeast, where you seldom notice it. But it's still there, trashing your health. This is one of the reasons I eat open-faced sandwiches with one slice of bread—an open-faced sandwich limits the sodium (as well as concentrated calories). I encourage you to do the same thing during the course of the Seven-Day Rescue. Check out the "Building Your Rescue Flats" section on pages 217–227.

Another huge source of sodium: restaurant food. The latest data from the trade publication *Restaurants and Institutions* reveals that millennials eat out an average of 3.4 times per week, Generation Xers 2.5 times per week, boomers 2.3 times per week, and as soon as Generation Zers begin earning money, their average will likely exceed millennials'.

Successful restaurants require repeat customers, so they dump as much salt as they can into their food to make it addictively tasty. For example, stop by Burger King for a bacon-and-cheese Whopper, and you'll take in 1,390 mg of sodium! Add a serving of large fries to that Whopper, and you're at 2,070 mg! Take a stroll into a TGI Fridays and gobble down the "healthy" Chipotle Yucatan Chicken Salad, and you've earned yourself 1,420 mg of sodium. Add the avocado vinaigrette dressing, and you've now topped the salt scales at 1,990 mg. Meanwhile, step inside the Macaroni Grill and have their Classic Italian Bake and get ready to pull out your blood pressure medication on the spot: You've just knocked back 4,890 mg of sodium. Hey, the Dead Sea called, they want their salt back!

The Worst Salt Offenders

According to the CDC, the top ten contributors of sodium to our diets are:

Bread and rolls—7.4 percent
Cold cuts/cured meats—5.1 percent
Pizza—4.9 percent
Fresh and processed poultry—4.5 percent
Soups—4.3 percent
Sandwiches, including cheeseburgers—4.0 percent
Cheese—3.8 percent
Pasta dishes like spaghetti with meat sauce—3.3
    percent
Meat dishes like meat loaf with tomato sauce—3.2
    percent
Snacks, including chips, pretzels, popcorn, and
    puffs—3.1 percent

So how do you best avoid the salt trap? Try to eat whole, plant-based foods that don't come in a package or a box. However, when you do eat packaged or boxed foods, you'll want to follow these label-reading rules and guidelines. I was taught these from the brilliant dietician Jeff Novick, whom we met in chapter 2.

The first guideline when looking at any package, box, or canned product? Never, ever believe any of the health claims. It's all just marketing mumbo jumbo.

Instead, look at the nutrition facts panel on the back. Here is Jeff's simple rule: If the milligrams of sodium are more than the calories per serving, leave it on the shelf. In other words, the ratio of sodium to calories should be no more than 1:1. Most soups, pasta sauces, and canned goods have anywhere from three to ten times more milligrams of sodium than calories per serving. Classic all-American Campbell's Tomato Soup, for example, has 90 calories and 480 mg of sodium.

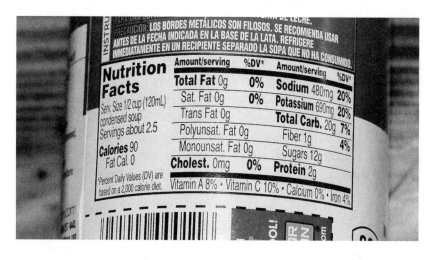

How about we leave the Campbell's for Andy Warhol and we'll eat some healthy soup like the Miso Barley on page 230.

Next up, a box of P. Terry's veggie burgers: They may be a svelte 220 calories per patty, but don't let your eyes bulge out of your head when you see the 580 mg of sodium! A bottle of Newman's Own marinara pasta sauce has a scant 70 calories per serving, but also an artery-scorching 460 mg of sodium! Pick up a can of Bush's Black Beans at 100 calories per serving, and you'll find nothing less than 490 mg of heart-stopping sodium!

Dumping in salt is the cheapest way to give these products maximum shelf life, to give them flavor without putting in more expensive spices and herbs, and, most important, to make you a regular customer. If you follow Jeff's 1:1 rule, within ten seconds you can determine if a product belongs in your grocery cart or the Dumpster.

Meanwhile, as long as you eat whole-food, plant-based meals, you'll never take in too much sodium. If your diet follows the Engine 2 guidelines, during the course of the Seven-Day Rescue Diet you should be getting no more than 500 mg of naturally occurring sodium per day from your plant-strong food, and another 500 to 1,000 mg from condiments, sauces, and packaged and canned foods.

For example, a cup of spinach has 24 mg of natural sodium. A medium apple has 2 mg of sodium. A large potato has 42 mg, a half cup of brown rice has 5 mg, and a cup of grilled portabella mushrooms has

13 mg of sodium. With delicious plant-strong foods, the Seven-Day Rescue program has been able to bring people's blood pressure down by an average of 10/5 mm/Hg, and some by as much as 60/40.

Read labels following Jeff's 1:1 guideline; don't cook with salt; lightly salt your food; eat whole, strong, plant-based foods; and watch as your blood pressure drops and your taste buds come to life.

Once you dump the salt, instead of tasting nothing but sodium you'll savor the natural scrumptiousness of sweet brown rice, a fresh bunch of steamed broccoli with lemon juice, or a Cara Cara orange.

SUGAR

Our country suffers from a major, intense, powerful sweet tooth. The latest data indicate that on average Americans consume nearly *30 teaspoons* of added sugar a day. In case you were wondering, according to the American Heart Association, the suggested upper limit is 9 teaspoons of added sugar for men and 6 teaspoons for women.

During the Seven-Day Rescue, we will keep added teaspoons of sugar closer to 1 or, better yet, 0. And don't worry, your food will be juicy, succulent, flavorsome, and scrumptious!

White sugar, brown sugar, corn syrup, molasses, sucrose, fructose, sorbitol: The issue isn't what kind of added sweetener is the best or the worst. The issue is that people are completely overdosing on sweetness, no matter what it is. In fact, most people are now consuming nearly 160 pounds of added sugars per person, per year! (At the dawn of the American Revolution in 1776, we consumed just 4 pounds.) Frankly, I'm not interested in what type of sugar you're using. They all contain roughly 50 calories per tablespoon and they are metabolized in the same unpleasant way.

The bottom line is that Americans are pouring on added sugars like there is no tomorrow, and, consequently, many of us have a lot fewer tomorrows. Indeed, a study from the School of Medicine at the University of California, San Francisco, published in the *American Journal of Public Health*, concluded that added sugars have been linked to telomere shortening. Telomeres are the caps at the end of each strand of DNA. Picture the cap on the end of a shoelace. These little items have many tasks, including protecting our genetic data and regulating our aging process. When in good shape, telomeres keep chromosome ends from fraying, preventing DNA damage. Think of telomeres like a bomb fuse: The shorter your telomeres get, the less time you have to live. It turns out that people who drink 20 ounces a day of sugar-sweetened beverages have shorter telomeres than those who don't. In fact, they are so much shorter, researchers have predicted that these sugar-guzzlers will ultimately lose five years of life.

Interestingly, the only scientific data supporting the *lengthening* of telomeres was done by Dr. Dean Ornish at the University of California, San Francisco, in conjunction with Dr. Elizabeth Blackburn, who won the Nobel Prize for her work on the telomere. Dr. Ornish performed this feat with a group of men following a whole food, plant-based diet over a three-month period, during which Dr. Ornish successfully showed the ability of plants to stop and reverse prostate cancer.

In addition, added sugars hit your digestive system like a freight train. In response, your body immediately pumps out insulin to deal with all that excess blood sugar. In the hours following, you actually become hypoglycemic, which means all that insulin has actually made your blood sugar too *low*. The only option remaining for your body is to dump fat into your bloodstream to get things under control. This added fat creates a constant level of inflammation and contributes to many of the chronic Western diseases including heart disease, diabetes, cancer, obesity, metabolic syndrome, and autoimmune disorders.

Naturally occurring sugars, however, like those found in berries, kiwi, eggplant, quinoa, butternut squash, and pinto beans, do not cause these blood sugar and insulin spikes. This is largely due to the high fiber content of whole-plant foods. Fiber—which is found only in plants— has a wonderful gelling effect that not only makes you feel nice and full, but also binds to sugar and slows down the rate at which it is absorbed into your blood.

There is almost no limit to how much naturally occurring sugar you can eat! These sugars represent your body's primary fuel source, and you do not want to shy away from them. For example, even though a large banana contains more than 15 grams of natural sugar, we let it slip because fructose in a banana is attached to nearly 4 grams of fiber. But remember, when you remove sugar from its fiber—which happens when you juice—you lose most of the health benefits. (For more information, see chapter 3.)

I recently came across a fantastic article in the *American Journal of Clinical Nutrition* that broke down how fiber works its magic. In a study that took place at the University of Eastern Finland's Institute of Public Health and Clinical Nutrition, one group of participants drank both a glass of sugar water and a glass of berry juice. A second group drank the sugar water and then ate a bunch of actual berries. Predictably, within fifteen minutes the juice group experienced a massive blood sugar spike. But among the berry group, despite consuming the same amount of sugar overall, there was no such spike. The soluble fiber in the berries was even able to neutralize the additional sugar water, and the result was no insulin shock and no inflammation-promoting fat dumped into the blood.

Unfortunately, too many people think that added sugars are just empty calories, that they provide no nutrition but aren't overtly bad for us as long as we consume them in moderation. Here we go again, folks: that dreaded M-word. Remember, moderation is *not* your friend. Moderation is the enemy. Moderation is saying: "Hey, I'll eat only a *moderate amount* of poison that is making me sick and stealing away years of good health." To that I say: "Not during the Seven-Day Rescue!"

Added sugars are added poison. Simple as that. Apart from piling on weight, added sugars can lead to chronic disease. Let's start with liver toxicity. Added sugars in the form of fructose—from sodas, pastries, and juices, to name a few—overload your liver's ability to process them into energy. As a result, much of the sugar is converted into pure fat, which finds its way into your bloodstream as LDL—"the bad"—cholesterol. As we know, this leads to inflammation in your arteries. But globs of fat also pile up in the liver, leading to an increasingly common condition known as nonalcoholic fatty liver disease. Just like with alcoholics, sugarholics also damage their livers, too often fatally. Meanwhile, as a 2013 study in the *Journal of Hepatology* concluded, "Industrial, not fruit fructose intake is associated with the severity of liver fibrosis." In other words, natural sugars found in whole fruits are perfectly healthy, while added sugars promote liver scarring.

Is Sugar Addictive?

As you were growing up, your mom may have told you to lay off the Froot Loops and Count Chocula because you'd get hooked on the sugar. Was that an old wives' tale? Or is all that added sugar truly addictive?

Well, your mom was onto something, even though she probably didn't have access to multimillion-dollar PET scan machines back in the day. A 2011 analysis published in *Trends in Cognitive Sciences* explained how sophisticated brain scanners reveal that obese individuals have decreased dopamine sensitivity, just as alcohol and drug addicts do. Dopamine is a chemical neurotransmitter that helps trigger pleasure in the brain. As the renowned clinical psychologist Vaughan Bell quips, dopamine is the "Kim Kardashian of neurotransmitters." It's released during pleasurable activities and can motivate someone to seek out that activity again and again. Sex, drugs, alcohol, and, it turns out, eating, can each stimulate dopamine, which also explains why we can become addicted to those things. Once dopamine receptors in the brain become desensitized, more and more sex, drugs, booze, or food is necessary for a satisfactory amount of pleasure.

This latest study suggests that sugar, like sex and drugs, might well play a major role in food addiction and overeating. As we pile on the sugar, we need more and more of it to derive pleasure from eating. When you consider that nearly 80 percent of all food in the American food supply contains added sugars, you'd wonder if the food companies knew about this long before the scientists!

Meanwhile, salt isn't the only little white crystal that promotes high blood pressure. A 2014 analysis published in the journal *Open Heart* determined that added sugars play "a major role in the development of hypertension." Among studies lasting eight weeks or more, high sugar intake was found to boost systolic blood pressure by 6.9 mm/Hg and diastolic blood pressure by 5.6 mm/Hg. Meanwhile, people who consume 25 percent or more of their calories from added sugars have triple the risk of death from cardiovascular disease. And good old fruit? As a review in the journal *Diabetes* points out, "Whereas fructose from added sugars is associated with hypertension, fructose from natural fruits is not."

I feel like I am in control. Food doesn't control me. I actually LOVE what I eat. I look forward to my oatmeal with fruit in the morning and my veggie burgers on whole-wheat wraps. And, of course, all the fruit and vegetables and whole grains—it's all so great! I don't miss anything from before. Not sugar, not cheese, not meat.
                                    —Bruno Giannini, age 55, event planner

Whether you're chugging a soda, lapping up a Greek yogurt, or spooning cereal, I'll bet you dollars to donuts that you're consuming sugar beyond your wildest dreams. For example, that 12-ounce can of Coke you're downing as an afternoon pick-me-up boasts 10 teaspoons of sugar. Your daily Greek yogurt with fruit, which claims to have zero fat and enough protein to get you sprinting out the door in the morning, has between 4 and 5 teaspoons of added sugar. That box of Honey Nut Cheerios your kids scream for before running out to catch the school bus has 2 added teaspoons of sugar per serving. Meanwhile, that post-workout Snickers bar boasts 7 teaspoons, and you'll find 15 teaspoons of sugar in that innocent Jamba Juice Banana Berry Smoothie!

We have to outfox the food manufacturers by beating them at their own game. To do this, it's crucial to differentiate between naturally occurring sugars, which are healthy, and added sugars, which are not.

Again, let's use Jeff Novick's label-reading guidelines, but this time for sugar. The easiest way is to look at the ingredients list and see how many types of sugars are listed and where they fall in the list. First of all, we don't want to eat a product that has sugar listed as one of the first three ingredients. (Remember, ingredients have to be listed in descending order by the weight.) If sugar is listed as one of the first three ingredients, leave that cavity bomb on the shelf.

Second, we don't want to eat a product that has more than three kinds of added sugars. You'll be dumbfounded when you discover that some of your favorite products have five to ten different types of sugar! It's super simple and fun when you can shop the aisles and see right through manufacturers' attempts to sweeten you up. Sometimes they try to use sophisticated names to conceal what that impostor sugar really is, so be sure to look out for anything that says "evaporated cane juice syrup," "evaporated cane juice," "agave nectar," "molasses," "beet sugar," "malt," "barley malt," "cane juice crystals," "corn sweetener," "corn syrup," "ethyl maltol," and the evil granddaddy of them all, "high-fructose corn syrup."

What's in Your Cereal?

Here's the ingredient list for seemingly healthy Fiber One Honey Clusters—all of the different kinds of sugar are highlighted. Count them!

Ingredients: Whole Grain Wheat, Corn Bran, Wheat Bran, Chicory Root Extract, Whole Grain Oats, Crisp Oats (Rice Flour, Whole Grain Oats, **Sugar, Malt Extract**), Toasted Oats (Whole Grain Oats, **Sugar, High Fructose Corn Syrup**, Soybean Oil, **Honey, Brown Sugar, Molasses**), Salt, Wheat Bits (Whole Grain Wheat, Corn Starch, Corn Flour, **Sugar**, Salt, Trisodium Phosphate, Baking Soda, Color Added), **Barley Malt Extract, Honey**, Modified Corn Starch, **Malt**

Syrup, Tripotassium Phosphate, Color Added, Cinnamon, Natural And Artificial Flavor, **Sucralose**, Walnut Meal, Almond Meal, Nonfat Milk. Vitamin E (Mixed Tocopherols) And BHT Added To Preserve Freshness. Vitamins And Minerals: Calcium Carbonate, Zinc And Iron (Mineral Nutrients), Vitamin C (Sodium Ascorbate), A B Vitamin (Niacinamide), Vitamin B_6 (Pyridoxine Hydrochloride), A B Vitamin (Folic Acid), Vitamin B_{12}.

So in this box of Fiber One cereal there are *twelve* different kinds of sugar listed all over the ingredients panel! Do not go anywhere near this abomination! If you want fiber, get it straight from the source: fruits, vegetables, legumes, and whole grains.

Can Diabetics Eat Fruit?

There's another misconception out there that people who are suffering from type 2 diabetes or prediabetes should avoid fruit due to its sugar content. Not only is this wrong, it's dangerous. Consuming lots of fruit can actually *slow down* and *reverse* the progression of type 2 diabetes.

This was proved in a superb pilot study published in the *Open Journal of Preventive Medicine*. Thirteen diabetic men and women were switched over from a typical Western diet to a plant-strong diet replete with greens, sumptuous veggies, whole grains, legumes, and seeds. Moreover, they had fruit with each and every meal. After seven months, the participants' A1C levels—a measure of how well your body is controlling blood sugar—dropped from an average of 8.2 to a nondiabetic

> 5.8. Amazingly, during the trial, many of the participants stopped taking their blood sugar–lowering medications altogether.
>
> During our Engine 2 Seven-Day Rescue camps, I routinely have people coming off their insulin and cutting their oral medications in half (with the supervision of our medical director) in just seven days! Doctors might call this a miracle, but we know better. It's not a miracle. This is the reality of what can happen when you put strong, whole, plant-based foods into your body on a consistent basis.

FAT

Fat. We are fat. Very fat. According to the CDC, 75 percent of Americans are now considered either overweight or obese. One big reason: We eat too much fat itself, most of which comes from animals and refined oils. For many people, unnecessary and unhealthy fats represent more than 33 percent of their total calorie intake. This overconsumption of weak fats is a major contributing factor to the pool of diseases that are fattening up our bottoms along with our annual health-care bills.

There are three types of fat: trans fats, saturated fats, and unsaturated fats. Trans fats are the meanest, ugliest, artery-clogging, heart-stopping villains of them all. They occur in *all* meat and dairy products, and they appear in packaged and boxed foods as partially hydrogenated oils. Hydrogenation is a chemical process whereby hydrogen is added to liquid oils to turn them solid, which increases a product's shelf life and decreases your shelf life. These fats are Bad news with a capital *B*: Research from the Harvard School of Public Health concludes that trans fats are horrendous for your health even in tiny doses: for every 2 percent of your daily calories that come from trans fat, your risk of heart disease skyrockets by 23 percent!

These are the fats that were banned in all New York City restaurants in 2006, and more recently from all packaged foods since they no longer meet the FDA's distinction of being "generally recognized as safe" for human consumption. The food industry has until 2018 to remove artificial trans fats from all processed food products, but you can get a jump start and avoid these products even before they're pulled from the shelves by understanding how to read labels. Be careful, though. Food manufacturers are very clever. Their products can still contain trans fat even if the ingredients panel says "zero trans fat." If you spot any ingredients that say "partially hydrogenated oil," or if it includes margarine, or if you see the term "shortening," there are trans fats. Toss them out of your shopping cart and onto the Trans-Siberian Railway!

Next up, fats that are solid at room temperature are known as saturated fats, and they are found almost exclusively in meat and dairy products. The only exceptions are nuts and seeds (5 to 10 percent saturated fat) and coconuts (91 percent). During the next seven days, I want you to steer clear of saturated fats because of their association with promoting heart disease, type 2 diabetes, major cancers, and obesity. If people tell you they are a fan of saturated fats, what they're essentially saying is they're a fan of meat and dairy products. This is why the Atkins people, the South Beach people, and most recently the Paleo people are trying to bring back saturated fat. It's the lifeblood of their programs. Of course, if everyone had time to read the medical literature, all these gimmicky diets would be dead in the water. But people love to hear good news about their bad habits (remember those old ads from the 1950s claiming most doctors choose Camel cigarettes?) and will hang on until the bitter end.

Here's a Finnish study that really blew my mind. Right after World War II, Finland decided to jump on the meat-and-dairy bandwagon like the rest of the Western world. Sure enough, that wagon brought Finland to the same health wasteland it brought America. The Finnish diet was high in saturated-fat-laden meat and dairy products, heavy in salt, low in fruits and vegetables, and by the 1970s the mortality rate due to heart disease among Finnish men was the highest in the world. But a group of intrepid researchers decided to help convert Finnish dairy farmers into berry farmers, and eventually the project expanded into educating the entire country about the dangers of a diet based around saturated fat. It paid off. For instance, in 1972, 60 percent of Finns reported using butter on their bread. Nowadays, barely 5 percent do. Over the ensuing decades there was as much as an *80 percent drop* in heart disease mortality and a seven-year boost in life expectancy for men and a six-year boost for women. Not surprisingly, that coincided with a big drop in saturated fat intake, from 21 percent of total calories to 14 percent.

But the problems with saturated fat don't end with heart disease. The Harvard Women's Health Study, which followed thousands of women for ten years, concluded that high saturated-fat intake, mainly from the likes of processed foods, meat, and dairy, is associated with cognitive decline. Women who consumed the most saturated fat had 60 to 70 percent increased odds of experiencing deteriorated brain function, while those who took in the least saturated fat had the same brain function on average as women six years younger!

In addition, saturated fat can build up in muscle cells, which can lead to insulin resistance and type 2 diabetes. Moreover, saturated fat can also kill off the delicate beta cells in your pancreas that produce insulin. As a study from the University of Minnesota, reported in the *American Journal of Clinical Nutrition*, concluded, "The proportional saturated fatty acid composition of plasma is positively associated with the development of diabetes. Our findings...suggest indirectly that the dietary fat profile, particularly that of saturated fat, may contribute to the etiology of diabetes."

And listen up, fellas: When it comes to saturated fat, you need to worry about your johnson along with your ticker. A recent Harvard University study suggested that just a small increase in saturated-fat intake was associated with a significant drop in sperm count. Another study published in the *American Journal of Clinical Nutrition* found that consuming lots of saturated fat can reduce sperm counts by as much as 65 percent!

Let's keep this simple: If that fat comes from an animal, it should stay in the animal. Animal fats have fault lines the size of San Andreas. The fat from beef is nearly 40 percent saturated. Chicken fat is more than 30 percent saturated. Egg fat is more than 30 percent saturated. But the number one source of saturated fat isn't meat or eggs—it's dairy, specifically cheese. Yes, your beloved cheese! That concentrated source of cow milk is more than 80 percent fat (and 70 percent saturated). Did you know that whole milk is 51 percent fat? One 8-ounce glass has the same amount of saturated fat as 4 strips of bacon. Two percent milk is 35 percent fat, and one glass has the same amount of saturated fat as 2½ strips of bacon. And 1 percent milk is actually 25 percent fat and has the same amount of saturated fat as 1½ strips of bacon. (The percentages in milk refer to the amount of fat by *weight*, not by calories. For example, if you have 100 pounds of 2 percent milk, 2 pounds of the milk is pure fat.)

In addition to all the health problems associated with trans and saturated fats, there are also toxic heavy metals, pesticides, and pollutants that migrate to, and are stored in, the fat of animals. Dioxins, for example, are environmental pollutants that can cause reproductive and developmental disorders, destroy the immune system, and cause cancer. You don't get them from asbestos or insecticides, though: More than 90 percent of human exposure comes through eating saturated fats from meat, dairy, and fish.

Finally, there are two types of *un*saturated fat: monounsaturated and polyunsaturated. Monounsaturated oils are liquid at room temperature, but when refrigerated they begin to solidify. The biggest source of monounsaturated fats is cooking oils, especially canola, olive, and peanut; nuts such as macadamias and hazelnuts; and fatty vegetables such as olives and avocados. Monounsaturated fats are unnecessary, and research by Dr. Lawrence Rudel from the Wake Forest School of Medicine suggests that monounsaturated fats promote atherosclerosis at the same rate as saturated fats, much to the dismay of everyone who thinks a Mediterranean-style diet based on olive oil, olives, and avocados is healthy. (For more information about the dangers of cooking oil, see chapter 2.)

But don't despair! We've read all about *bad* fats, but there are good-guy fats out there as well! I'm talking about *poly*unsaturated fats. Not only are they healthy, they are essential. Your body cannot live without polyunsaturated fats, and that's why you need to be eating *more* of them! Like many other vital nutrients, your body cannot produce its own polyunsaturated fats—they must come from your food. More specifically, they must come from plant food. Once you realize there is an abundance of naturally occurring healthy fats in plant-based foods, you will never look at oats or kale the same way!

During the course of the Seven-Day Rescue, we'll be focusing on polyunsaturated fats, specifically omega-3 fatty acids. These fats help your body do pretty much every darn thing possible: fight infections, regulate blood clotting, build muscle, burn fat, preserve brain function, destroy cancer cells, and prevent heart disease and stroke by reducing inflammation and lowering blood pressure. The best sources of omega-3s are whole, plant-based foods such as green leafy vegetables, beans, ground flaxseed meal, walnuts, chia seeds, and hemp seeds.

The other type of polyunsaturated fats are omega-6 fatty acids, but these aren't nearly as healthy as omega-3s. In fact, most of us are getting more omega-6s than we should, mainly because these days omega-6s are overwhelmingly found in processed foods and vegetable oils. Throughout most of human evolution, our ratio of omega-3s to omega-6s was about 1:1. That's because we mainly ate plants, not Pringles. Nowadays, however, most Americans have anywhere from a 10:1 to a whopping 25:1 ratio of omega-6s to omega-3s. The science is complicated, but in short form, too many omega-6s in your diet can cancel out the health benefits of omega-3s. The result is chronic-disease-promoting inflammation.

You have to be careful with omega-6 fats because excessive amounts are found in certain plant foods. For example, almonds have a horrendous 2,500:1 ratio of omega-6s to omega-3s. That ain't going to cut the mustard during the Seven-Day Rescue. Instead, we're going to limit our nut intake to walnuts. They have the lowest ratio of omega-3s to omega-6s at 1:3, which will help alleviate the chronic inflammation that has built up in your body after years of eating the wrong foods.

During the Rescue Diet, your total calories from plant fats will top off at 15 percent—with 0 percent coming from animal fats. This will allow you to get plenty of nurturing and healthy essential omega fats while your body starts to heal itself at a cellular level and a macro level. In fact, my father insists that his patients who are reversing their heart disease derive no more than 10 percent of their calories from fat, and he has achieved some of the most dramatic before-and-after results in medical history.

In addition to limiting your intake of nuts, seeds, and avocados, you need to learn how to read a food label to determine how much fat resides in any given product. I'm a little more lenient than my father is, but we still want to make sure that no more than 25 percent of any packaged food's calories come from fat, just as I recommended in my first book, *The Engine 2 Diet.*

The nutrition facts label does most of the math for us—there's a handy "calories from fat" panel that helps us figure it out. Let's take Lay's Classic Potato Chips, for example. The total calories per serving are 160, but the calories from fat are a massive 90. The easiest way to figure out 25 percent, using simple division, is to look for the total calories per serving. Next, divide those calories by four—that will give your magical 25 percent. For example, in our Lay's potato chips, the total calories are 160. If we divide by 4, we get 40. Therefore, we don't want our calories from fat to be over 40. With the Lay's, the number of calories coming from fat is 90, which is definitely greater than 40. So give those chips the ol' heave-ho!

If you do the math and divide 90 by 160, you'll discover the amount of fat in these potato chips is actually 56 percent, unlike, say, a delicious baked sweet potato, which has 60 calories but only 1 lonely calorie from fat—good for an artery-soothing 1.6 percent.

Nutrition Facts

Serving Size 1 oz (28g/About 15 chips)
Servings Per Container 10

Amount Per Serving

Calories 160	Calories from Fat 90

	% Daily Value*
Total Fat 10g	**16%**
Saturated Fat 1.5g	**8%**
Trans Fat 0g	
Cholesterol 0mg	**0%**
Sodium 170mg	**7%**
Potassium 350mg	**10%**
Total Carbohydrate 15g	**5%**
Dietary Fiber 1g	**5%**
Sugars less than 1g	
Protein 2g	

Another task I want you to undertake when you are buying packaged, canned, and boxed goods: Read the list of ingredients and be on the lookout for added fats we want to avoid over the next seven days. These include saturated animal fats such as butter, eggs, lard, cheese, chicken fat, and beef fat; trans fats in the form of partially hydrogenated and hydrogenated vegetable oils; and all extracted vegetable oils such as olive oil, canola oil, sunflower oil, safflower oil, grape-seed oil, coconut oil, palm oil, corn oil, flaxseed oil, and walnut oil.

Plants are the mother lode of healthy fats. Did you know that *all* plant-based foods contain essential fats? Strawberries, apples, potatoes, corn, and even grapes all have fat just like they have protein and carbohydrates—and without any of the disease-promoting garbage you get with animal-based food. Simple oats? Sixteen percent fat. Kale? Eleven percent fat. Grapes? Nine percent fat.

When you load up on healthy fats, your body will thank you. Your cells will become liberated, your mind will become clear, your heart will sing, and your libido will reach new heights!

What About Fish Oil Supplements?

There's a lot of fishy science out there claiming that we can get all the healthy omega-3 fatty acids we need from pills stuffed with processed fish oil. What's up with this, and who would ever try such a thing?

Well, it turns out a lot of people do. Americans now consume upward of 100,000 tons of fish oil every year.

Is it doing any good? No! This whole fish oil nonsense began in the 1980s when one study published in the *Lancet* found that men might see a reduction in heart disease mortality if they took fish oil pills. Of course everyone seems to forget the follow-up study, run by the same group of researchers, which found that fish oil pills could actually *promote* heart disease! And recent studies haven't been any kinder. A major review published in the *Journal of the American Medical Association* looked at all the best randomized trials and concluded that fish oil supplementation "was not associated with a lower risk of all-cause mortality, cardiac death, sudden death, myocardial infarction, or stroke."

Nevertheless, the American Heart Association continues to advise people with a history of heart disease to ask their doctor about fish oil supplements despite their dubious benefits. Indeed, a review published in the *Archives of Internal Medicine* found "insufficient evidence of a secondary preventive effect of omega-3 fatty acid supplements against overall cardiovascular events among patients with a history of cardiovascular disease."

I've said it before and I'll say it again: Fish oil is just snake oil. Don't try it!

We are drowning in seas of salt, lakes of sugar, and oceans of fat. Instead of sending us life vests, the food companies are sending us lead weights. When you hear about conglomerates like Unilever investing $30 million in a twenty-person team to study the sensory power of high-fat food—or when soda companies use regression analysis and sophisticated math to find the "bliss point," that ideal amount of salt, sugar, and fat to add to their product for peak addiction—you realize that multibillion-dollar corporations don't always have our best interests in mind.

Your body wants to fight back against salt, sugar, and fat. As a study in the *Journal of Food Science* points out, we can actually taste fat like we taste salt and sugar, and eating too much of all three blunts our taste buds. Like a drug addict, we need more and more to be satisfied.

The Seven-Day Rescue stops your addiction in its tracks. Once you lay off the added poisons, your taste buds actually become more sensitive again. I've had people come up to me after the seven days astounded by how much less salt they're pouring onto their food. This helps explain why a study published in the *American Journal of Clinical Nutrition* found that participants who switched to a low-salt diet for only a few weeks refused to return to heavily salted food. It tasted terrible!

I had a very difficult time with cravings the first few days of the Rescue Week. I craved salt and cheese A LOT. I felt very hungry before meals. However, as the week went on I stopped craving salt and cheese and meat. They started to seem kind of gross to me. I started to crave things like apples and Ezekiel 4:9 bread instead of pizza and candy!

—Jackie Plantner, age 38, school principal

Healthy, plant-based food tastes wonderful. If you've grown up on the typical American diet, you just need to give your poor taste buds some time to wake up. They've been beaten unconscious by the onslaught of salt, sugar, and fat. But don't worry, after seven days they will wake up with a vengeance, craving strong, healing plants!

7

Why We Exercise

Wait...what? Exercise? What does the Seven-Day Rescue Diet have to do with exercise? It says "diet" right there in the title. You're thinking: *Bring me back to the food, man! That part was fun!* After all, it's not called the Engine 2 Seven-Day Sweat Yourself to Death program. I once had an Engine 2 Rescue participant flat out tell me she would not engage in any type of exercise. No thank you, no sirree. The thought of exercise made her want to lie down and take a nap.

Well, I told her exactly what I am telling you: It's time! During the Rescue Week you are going to exercise, and I am convinced you will like it. And I know your body will. Why? Because not only is it good for you, it will make you feel better.

Just as proper diet is a pillar of good health, so is exercise.

From Ironman triathlons to mixed martial arts to mountaineering, the human body is capable of spectacular physical feats. But you don't need highly tuned genetics to be an athlete. Robust physical ability is encoded in everyone's DNA. Our ancestors routinely trekked, ran, and climbed many miles every day, and today we're designed to do exactly the same—even if these days the farthest we walk is to the mailbox.

What do most of us do? We get up in the morning and sit at the table for breakfast, sit in the car on the way to work, sit at a desk for eight hours, sit in the car again, sit at the table for dinner before sitting down to surf the Internet and then watch television. Then we lie down. The next day, we start the whole process all over again. Meanwhile, our children are even worse off: According to the Kaiser Family Foundation, the average American youth spends 7.5 hours every single day in front of a screen and just 7 minutes in the great outdoors. It seems the only time we're on our feet is when we're looking for a new place to sit. And have you seen these new motorized scooters and hoverboards that kids are now sporting? We are enabling a whole new generation to become even more sedentary and less fit.

This is troublesome.

Why? Because sitting has become the new smoking. As we'll read about in this chapter, study after study reveals just how dangerous it is for us to not move our bodies regularly. Our sedentary inertia has become a blanket of sticky molasses gluing us to our couches, and it's slowly killing us. According to research published in the *Lancet*, if Americans collectively exercised enough to reduce our body mass index (BMI) by just 1 measly percent, we could prevent 127,000 cases of cancer, 1.5 million cases of heart disease, and 2 million cases of diabetes!

I will do anything it takes to get your heart pumping, your lungs singing, and your muscles flexing. During our Seven-Day Rescue programs in the red canyons of Sedona, Arizona, it's mandatory for participants to sign up for an hour-long morning walk, an hour-long beginners' yoga class, or an hour-long CrossFit-type class that includes resistance training. By the end of the program, everyone builds wonderful new relationships with their bodies, awakening athletic abilities that had been dormant for years—or even decades.

During the first day's orientation session, when everyone is anxious and wondering to themselves, *What in the world have I gotten myself into?*, I explain that in addition to eating the most delicious, nutritious, and healing food on the planet, the participants will be rediscovering their own bodies. We offer daily afternoon hikes on some of the most amazing trails in the world, and first thing in the morning, everyone— and I mean *everyone*—participates in one of the workout options offered from 6:15 to 7:15. I've led eleven of these retreats, and sleeping in is not an option. In order to seal the deal, we take a vote. I ask people, "If you decide to sleep in while everyone else is sweating and working out, will you agree to come up to the front of the room and explain to everyone else why you slept in?" Every group has agreed!

Oh, we've had some wild excuses. I remember one person in particular who offered a little too much information. I had asked the group if anyone had missed their morning workout. A very sweet woman raised her hand, and without so much as batting an eye said: "I was heading over to yoga class, but I pooped my pants and had to regroup." We applauded her honesty. But barring any intestinal malfunctions, regular exercise in the morning will light a fire under your productivity, your spirit—and yes, your butt—for the rest of the day!

Of course, not everyone has the luxury of waking up in the gorgeous mountains of Sedona with a group of 100 people motivated to improve their quality of life. And you probably won't have a crazy guy like me barking at you at 6:00 a.m. to get your rear end out of bed! But don't worry. Exercise can become as habitual as brushing your teeth or putting on your seat belt. It'll take a little bit of work, but just like eating plant-strong, being body-strong is paramount for good mental and physical health.

> I woke up and just couldn't keep from exercising. Instead of driving to a friend's house, I put my kids in the stroller and walked the three-plus miles to her house. On Memorial Day I took my kids to the zoo and there wasn't parking nearby. I walked over a mile from where I ended up parking so that I could take them. Not long ago I would have just given up and left.
> —Karyn Blake, age 36, lawsuit production supervisor

What's the Big Deal with Sitting?

I know what you're thinking: *Yeah, yeah, our ancestors had to walk fifteen miles through blizzards and hurricanes just to reach that measly berry patch. We were a lot tougher back then, big deal. Nowadays we have Uber and scooters! Why walk when we can ride and roll?*

It's true that getting places is easier than ever, but it turns out that we humans don't rely on exercise just to get where we're going—we rely on exercise to stay alive. The first inklings of this connection arrived during the 1950s, when British researchers found that (constantly sitting) bus drivers in London were much more likely to suffer heart attacks compared to (constantly walking) ticket collectors. But today the evidence is overwhelming.

For example, the journal *Circulation* published a study of nearly 10,000 adults followed for seven years, determining that every extra hour spent watching TV per day is linked with an 11 percent increased chance of dying prematurely. Moreover, a fourteen-year American Cancer Society study of 100,000 Americans concluded that men who sit for six hours per day—whether on the couch, in the car, at work, or anywhere else—have a 20 percent higher rate of death compared to men who sit for three hours or less. Women who sit for more than six hours have a *40 percent* greater rate of death than women sitting for under three hours. Meanwhile, a massive analysis of nearly 800,000 people out of England's University of Leicester found that compared to individuals who are the most active, the biggest couch potatoes have a 112 percent increased risk of diabetes, 90 percent increased risk of fatal heart disease, and a 49 percent increased risk of death from any cause.

And don't think hitting the gym every day is going to help if you still spend most of the day on your tush. An analysis of more than forty studies published in the *American Journal of Preventive Medicine* determined that no matter how intensely you beat yourself up in the gym, spending too much of your time on your butt is still associated with a shorter life span. Similarly, as a study in the *American Journal of Epidemiology* noted, even if you bust your tail swimming or running for an hour every single day, sitting for another six hours still increases your chances of dying prematurely.

Why? After sitting for more than an hour, your body halts production of the fat-burning enzyme lipase by as much as 90 percent. This slows down the rate at which glucose is metabolized and lowers levels of HDL—"the good"—cholesterol. Your blood sugar rises, your muscles tighten, and the muscles in your legs don't sufficiently contract to send blood back up to your heart. As a result, excess blood pools in your legs, your cells clump together, and circulation slows. You start feeling tired—that's because your body is no longer producing enough insulin to ferry glucose to your muscles. Then you feel hungry, even if you just ate—this is because the appetite-regulating hormones leptin and ghrelin are completely out of whack. You eat more, you move less, and a vicious cycle ensues.

Improving Circulation at Work

Let's face it: Humans were not designed to have nine-to-five jobs. But as much as I'd love you to quit your job and come running with me down in Austin, I don't want you jeopardizing your family's financial well-being. Don't fret, though—if you work in an office all day, there is good news out of Indiana University.

The researchers first confirmed what we already knew: Extended sitting is very, very bad. They asked a group of healthy men to sit still without moving and, sure enough, found that their arteries' ability to pump blood was restricted by 50 percent within an hour. However, when the participants took a five-minute walk once an hour, their circulation returned to normal.

While sitting for most of the day is still not preferable, you can do your body a favor by walking over to your coworker's desk instead of e-mailing her, or taking the long way to the printer. Better yet, consider switching to a standing desk. Simply standing at work instead of sitting can raise your heart rate and burn off an extra 50 calories per hour. That comes out to an additional 30,000 calories per year—that's the same as if you ran ten marathons!

We need to get up and get moving. Lack of physical activity has now reached number four on the global causes-of-death list, right after high blood pressure, smoking, and high blood sugar. But you don't have to run ultramarathons to reap the benefits of exercise. For example, research presented at the 2015 European Society of Cardiology conference in London suggested that just taking a brisk twenty-five-minute walk every day can tack on three to seven years of extra life. Moreover, a Cambridge University research team tracking 300,000 Europeans for twelve years determined that daily walks reduced the death rate of normal-weight people by 25 percent, and by 16 percent among the obese.

Besides extending your life, there are plenty of additional reasons to have a nurturing relationship with your body and stay fit. Here are my top nine.

Exercise Improves Your Mood

That's right! Lift weights to lift your spirit! I don't know if there is a better mood enhancer or antidepressant on the planet than exercise. When you exercise, your body produces hormones called endorphins that immediately improve your mood. My wife, Jill, swims regularly with the local Masters swim program, primarily for the mood boost. If someone asks to pass her in the lane, she'll say: "Sure! I'm just here to get my endorphins flowing!"

If I can't incorporate a 30-minute bicycle ride, a 45-minute swim, or a 10-minute run into my day, I immediately feel my mood drop. But if I can get that swim, if I can leave the keys on the table and bike to the office, or if I manage a run with the dogs before dinner, I light up like a Roman candle. I'm as centered as the equator. I'm ready for anything life throws at me.

Science agrees with me! For example, a study out of Columbia University involving nearly 5,000 people found that those who regularly exercise have a 25 percent lower chance of being diagnosed with major depression. In another study, Duke University researchers randomly assigned depressed men and women either to take the antidepressant Zoloft or to try an aerobic exercise program. After four months, the exercise-only group improved at the same rate as the drug group—without the nasty side effects, which can include decreased libido in up to 75 percent of users, confusion, diarrhea, weight gain, drowsiness, lack of energy...the list is so endless it's, well, depressing. Compare that to the side effects of exercise: increased pleasure, weight loss, improved physical appearance, and longer life.

About three years ago, my wife and I were both close to morbidly obese. I was 320 pounds, she was—well, I know better than to tell a woman's weight. We decided it was time to change, and we started a workout program. We lost some weight (I lost about 30 pounds), but we slowly began gaining it back as we stopped working out. I had injured myself and Zita had stopped her exercise. With my injuries, I didn't want to stick to our outlined diet so we both ended up back to our old ways.

I had managed to take more weight off, but it always came back as I would end a program or get too busy with work. Then, close to two years ago, we saw *Forks over Knives* on Netflix. We had no idea what it was about, but it sounded interesting. After our viewing, we decided to give it a try for a month—we figured, "What's the worst that can happen in thirty days?" We went all in: no cheese, no meat, no eggs. As we learned about oils we began cutting those out as well.

Without exercise, we both started dropping weight. Slowly, we got back into exercise, which has sped up the process. Today, I'm down to 199 and she's down to 80 total pounds lost. We stand today eating plant-strong and in great shape. We both still have weight to lose to get to our ideal weights, but that will come in time. For the first time we both see the light at the end of the tunnel, and knowing we can finally be in good shape is amazing. We don't plan to stop eating like this when we get there, either—this is a change we've committed to for the rest of our lives.

Thank you again, Rip, for all the work you do. It's truly an inspiration.

—Alex Winkler, age 34, traveling consultant; and
Zita Winkler, age 28, social worker

Moreover, it's not even clear if antidepressants work any better than a placebo. Big Pharma loves to tout the effectiveness of their drugs by publishing thousands of clinical trials, but they don't like to tell us about the unpublished trials—you know, the ones that show their drugs are no better than sugar pills. According to an analysis in the *New England Journal of Medicine*, when you factor in unpublished studies it turns out that *half* of all trials conclude that drugs are useless at treating depression. This suggests that the placebo effect—the patient's expectation that a medication will be helpful—may largely account for the perceived benefits of antidepressants. (Keep in mind that these medications are beneficial for some people, so please make your decisions regarding drugs and therapy in consultation with your health specialists.)

Exercise regularly and you'll do what my family likes to call "getting out the oogies." Yes, that's an official medical term! My son, Kole, and my daughter Sophie have to get their oogies out on a daily basis with a nice swim in the pool, a bike ride, gymnastics, basketball, or soccer. Otherwise, they argue, fight, and are generally insufferable. It must run in the family, because Jill and I are the same way!

Yoga to Lift Your Mood

During the Seven-Day Rescue program, we encourage participants to try yoga. Not only is yoga great exercise, but it also has profound effects on your mental health. For example, a 2010 study out of Boston University found that just three weekly yoga sessions can boost your levels of GABA (gamma-aminobutyric acid), a brain chemical that is believed to improve mood and decrease anxiety.

In addition, a five-year study conducted by Dr. John Denninger, a psychiatrist at Harvard Medical School, suggests that mind-body yoga techniques can actually temporarily switch off genes associated with stress and anxiety. Finally, a study led by the Nobel Prize–winning biological researcher Elizabeth Blackburn found that regular meditation can reduce stress-induced aging by slowing the cellular aging process.

Namaste, y'all!

Exercise Improves Your Brain

In addition to strengthening your muscles, exercise also works out that big ol' mental muscle: your brain! When you exercise, your heart beats faster, which means more oxygen-rich blood is delivered to your brain. All that extra blood apparently pumps up an important region of the brain responsible for memory and learning. According to a study conducted at the University of British Columbia, regular aerobic exercise actually increases the size and effectiveness of the hippocampus, which scientists think is the center of emotion, memory, and the nervous system.

Exercise is able to reduce insulin resistance, reduce inflammation, and trigger the release of chemicals in your brain called growth factors, which govern the development and health of brain cells. As Harvard Medical School psychiatrist John Ratey states: "Exercise is the single best thing you can do for your brain in terms of mood, memory, and learning. Even ten minutes of activity changes your brain."

Exercise can be especially important for combating Alzheimer's disease and dementia. For example, in a recent two-year study, German researchers followed 4,000 people older than fifty-five and concluded that those who rarely exercised were more than twice as likely to experience cognitive decline compared to those who took part in active pursuits such as swimming, cycling, and gardening. Moreover, after tracking 1,500 people for twenty years, researchers published a study in the *Lancet Neurology* concluding that "regular physical activity may reduce the risk or delay the onset of dementia and [Alzheimer's disease], especially among genetically susceptible individuals." People who exercised at least twice per week during middle age were much less likely to experience cognitive decline in their sixties and seventies compared to people who did not exercise.

When it comes to exercise, remember what Dr. Ratey likes to say: "A sound mind lives in a healthy body."

Exercise Boosts Your Immune System

Out with the old and in with the new! When you exercise, you feed the 37 trillion cells in your body with wonderfully fresh, oxygenated blood, and you accelerate the dumping of waste products that are keeping you down and out. Throughout my athletic career I've noticed that fit people are also the least sick people, and science agrees 100 percent!

For example, a study published in the *British Journal of Sports Medicine* found that if you let your kids run around for just six minutes, the levels of infection-fighting immune cells circulating in their blood increases by 50 percent. Meanwhile, an Appalachian State University study concluded that while sedentary senior women have about a 50 percent chance of developing an upper-respiratory illness during the fall, those who take a daily thirty-minute walk have only a 20 percent chance of becoming sick, and those who run regularly have just an 8 percent chance. Likewise, a study published in the *American Journal of Medicine* found that women who took a thirty-minute walk every day for a year had half the number of colds as women who did not exercise. Finally, a study conducted by researchers at the University of Nebraska Medical Center and the Rocky Mountain Cancer Rehabilitation Institute demonstrated that the potency of T cells—key white blood cells that fight infection—improved drastically among cancer survivors who participated in a twelve-week exercise class.

And speaking of cancer, University of North Carolina at Chapel Hill researchers concluded in 2012 that regular exercise can reduce the risk of breast cancer. They found that both pre- and postmenopausal women who exercised between ten and nineteen hours per week had as much as a 30 percent decreased risk of developing breast cancer.

Exercise Boosts Your Appetite and Makes You Love Food

Exercise of any kind will naturally increase your appetite, which makes it much easier to snack on an orange, apple, plum, or pear. As a study published in the *Proceedings of the Nutrition Society* points out, our bodies have evolved to crave 3 calories of food for every 10 calories we burn.

This phenomenon is especially useful when you are just beginning your plant-strong journey. Your taste buds are still being weaned off all the salt, sugar, and fat that inundate the typical American diet, so when you're super hungry you can really appreciate the ability of plants to fill you up. If you aren't hungry for delicious brown rice, black beans, oatmeal, oranges, or beets, then you haven't yet given yourself the opportunity to get adequately hungry, or maybe you still have junk food lying around the house that's making it harder for you to reach for the healthier, whole-food, plant-strong options. In case of the latter, here's what you're going to do: Throw out all the Lay's, Cheetos, and Hot Pockets and go for a long walk or jog. Wait until you're nice and hungry, then whip up a simple plant-based meal like the Sloppy Joe Tostados on page 245. The hungrier you are, the more delicious plants will taste—and the more you'll want to eat them again and again. And remember, as we learned in chapter 4, due to their low calorie density, you can eat as many plant-strong foods as you want without worrying about gaining weight!

Don't laugh, but another benefit of exercise is that it makes going to the bathroom a heck of a lot easier. When you feel like you've got a logjam in there, one of the best things you can do is take your stool for a walk. I guarantee that within ten to fifteen minutes you'll be looking for a porcelain god in which to unload yourself so you can get on with your workout.

Beets: The Performance-Enhancing Vegetable

If you hang around professional athletes long enough, you'll hear about potent (and usually illegal) drugs some take to gain an edge. Steroids, testosterone, amphetamines, you name it. What if I told you there was a performance-enhancing food you could eat that's perfectly legal and extremely healthy? You don't even have to hire some shady dudes to score it for you. You can find it in the produce aisle of the grocery store!

I'm talking about beets. Yes, beets, those purple, rugged-looking vegetables that you normally don't look at twice. Well, it turns out that the unassuming beet has a trick up its stem: it's one of the best performance-enhancing foods around!

The title of this study says it all: "Whole beetroot consumption acutely improves running performance." Published in the *Journal of the Academy of Nutrition and*

Dietetics, researchers gave male and female athletes 1.5 cups of baked beets and then had them go for a 5K run. Sure enough, during the final mile the beet group pulled ahead of the control group, who were not given beets. It turns out that even though the beet dopers were running 5 percent faster than the control group by the end of the race, their hearts weren't pounding any harder. Similarly, other studies have found that beet juice can help free divers hold their breath for an extra thirty seconds due to improved oxygen efficiency. More power, less effort.

It turns out that the natural nitrates found in beets not only cause your arteries to dilate, which helps deliver more oxygen-rich blood to your muscles, but they also increase your body's ability to extract energy from oxygen. You don't have to be a finely tuned athlete to reap the benefits, though: if you are at risk of heart disease, beets have been shown in many studies to help reduce blood pressure.

So dope with beets for your health and for a personal record in a 5K, 10K, or marathon!

Exercise Lowers Your Risk of Osteoporosis

Exercise is extremely powerful when it comes to decreasing your chances of all forms of chronic Western illness, whether it's heart disease, cancer, dementia, type 2 diabetes, or obesity. Exercise can also ward off osteoporosis, a debilitating disease that causes bones to become so weak and brittle that even a mild fall or cough can cause fractures. According to the National Osteoporosis Foundation, 54 million Americans over the age of fifty suffer from osteoporosis and low bone density. This figure is expected to reach 71 million by 2030.

We've read about how the standard American diet is largely leading the charge for osteoporosis. In chapter 3 I mentioned a study published in the *BMJ* that followed more than 100,000 men and women for twenty years, revealing that dairy milk may actually *increase* your odds of bone and hip fracture. It turns out that eating animal products produces an unsafe acid load, forcing your body to leach calcium from its own bones to bring down the pH level. This sets you up for bone fractures later in life.

What to do? Beat back osteoporosis by adopting a plant-strong diet—and by breaking off that 24/7 relationship your butt has with your chair. Your bones are living structures. They need pressure and force applied to them in order to get stronger. Think of your bones as trees in the forest: The tallest and strongest trees became that way after years of growing and adapting to the wind and rain. The more they resist what nature throws at them, the stronger they grow. Likewise, you can strengthen your bones with weight-bearing exercises such as squats and yoga.

You don't even have to pump iron to pump up your bones: Just walking around your house with a weighted vest or a backpack can help. Don't laugh! Your bones will respond quickly to these exercises. Again, science agrees with me! For example, during a 2002 study, Mayo Clinic researchers found that premenopausal women who perform resistive back-strengthening exercises can increase bone mineral density in their lumbar spine, not to mention decrease their risk of bone fractures, compared to women who don't exercise. It's never too early to start, either: a study published in *BMC Medicine* found that "exercise can significantly enhance bone strength" among children.

Meanwhile, the more you challenge your bones, the stronger they get. A study of female college athletes published in the *Journal of Athletic Training* found that bone density was highest among those who participated in "high-impact" sports such as volleyball and basketball. But you don't have to sign up for that kickboxing tournament just yet: The *American Journal of Public Health* noted in a reported study that "men who jogged nine or more times per month had higher [bone mineral density] levels than those who jogged only one to eight times per month," and significantly higher bone density than men who never jogged at all.

Weight-bearing exercises are the best for your bones, but the science shows that almost all kinds of exercise can combat osteoporosis. And remember, plant-strong means bone-strong! When you combine exercise with the body-strengthening effects of eating strong food, the integrity and strength of your bones will never be better!

Exercise Increases Your Energy

That seems so counterintuitive, doesn't it? When you're feeling fatigued, do you really want to go for a long walk, run, or cycle? You probably think your tired carcass needs a nap, not a jog!

Actually, the best thing you can do when your body is feeling gassed is, well, give the couch the finger and step on the gas! By getting out there and accelerating your heart rate and pumping your 2.5 gallons of blood through your 65,000 miles of vessels, something magical happens. Your thoughts start expanding beyond work, your troubles seem distant, and you ignite an energy that gives you a lightness of being, a happy heart, and a glowing energy.

Think I'm crazy? Ask the team of researchers from the University of Georgia who pored through seventy separate studies on exercise and fatigue in nearly 7,000 people. The researchers concluded: "More than 90 percent of the studies showed the same thing: Sedentary people who completed a regular exercise program reported improved fatigue compared to groups that did not exercise." The analysis found that not only was exercise more effective than stimulant medications, but it can also boost energy levels among people suffering from chronic conditions such as heart disease and cancer.

If you can't step out for a jog, there is a simple breathing exercise you can perform to get recentered and relaxed. I call it the 7-7-7 exercise: Slowly breathe in for 7 seconds, hold it for 7 seconds, and then breathe out for 7 seconds. Then repeat it 7 times! The 7-7-7 exercise isn't as good as a hearty run, of course, but it gets your heart rate up to deliver oxygen-rich blood to wake up those lazy muscles!

A plant-strong diet gave me the ability to completely re-create myself from the inside out. I was able to change the way that I look, think, and feel through the food I was fueling myself with. Preparing a plant-based meal is very much an act of self-care and an act of self-love. It is saying that I choose to be a better version of myself today than the day before and I am choosing to promote health and wellness in my life.

—Adam Sud, age 33, lifestyle coach

Exercise Boosts Your Sex Life

Let's get real: When you feel good about how you look, you're more inclined to engage in some horizontal exercise. I've heard from countless people that once they complete the Engine 2 Rescue, they're amazed how much better they feel about their bodies—and how much better their sex lives have become. Much of this has to do with the "veggie Viagra effect"—namely, that a plant-strong diet improves blood flow not just to and from the heart, but to and from *everywhere*.

But exercise can have its own Viagra effect. For example, after following more than 600 middle-aged men for eight years, a team based out of the New England Research Institute found that regular exercise was extremely effective at lowering the risk of impotence. In another study, University of California, San Diego, researchers took about 80 healthy but sedentary men and asked some of them to begin exercise classes. By the end of the study, the researchers reported "significantly greater sexuality enhancements in the exercise group (frequency of various intimate activities, reliability of adequate functioning during sex, percentage of satisfying orgasms, etc.)."

Enough about men! Can women also see improvements in their sex lives from exercise? Yes! Researchers from my hometown of Austin, Texas, studied a group of women ages eighteen to thirty-four and concluded that vigorous exercise can improve blood flow to genital tissue and improve vaginal responses by as much as 169 percent.

So remember, folks, when it comes to sex, it's all about the blood flow. To improve your blood flow in bed, you first gotta get the blood flowing in the gym or on the track!

Exercise Makes It Easier to Get out of Bed in the Morning

Man, doesn't it feel horrible hitting that snooze button for the second, third, or fourth time every morning? Stumbling out of bed bleary-eyed is not the best way to start your day. It also doesn't help when you toss and turn every night, unable to fall asleep. I've had sleep problems like everyone else, but I've found that exercise helps me fall asleep within minutes. The moment the lights go off, so does my brain. But if I don't get in my daily jog, swim, or cycle, say good night to a good night's sleep!

Once again, science agrees! A study of more than 2,600 men and women published in the journal *Mental Health and Physical Activity* found that 150 minutes of moderate to vigorous exercise every week can provide a 65 percent boost in sleep quality. Moreover, participants who exercised reported feeling less sleepy, more productive, and were 68 percent less likely to experience leg cramps while sleeping and 45 percent less likely to have difficulty concentrating compared to people who did not exercise.

I learned a wonderful way to get up in the morning from one of our Seven-Day Rescue motivational speakers, Dick Beardsley, who is one of the greatest marathoners ever. Dick broke the Boston Marathon course record in 1982, and he holds the Guinness World Record for being the only man to ever run thirteen consecutive personal-best marathon times. Later in his career, after a number of serious car accidents and a brush with prescription-drug addiction, Dick developed a simple mental exercise that helped him get out of bed and through his day:

First, when you wake up, put a smile on your face. Hold it for several seconds. It's wild how your whole body reacts to a simple smile.

Second, strive to add enthusiasm in your voice when you speak. Anyone can walk around during the day with a monotone drone, but if you inject some gusto and spirit into your pipes, others will be inspired and you can spread the good energy.

Third, look for the joy in your heart. We all have it. Sometimes it may be hiding so well that you can't find it quickly, but if you really work, you'll locate it. When you do, bring it to the surface and add a joyous heart to your everyday personality.

Last, have faith in yourself. If you do, nothing nor anyone can take that away from you. Sure, we all have tough days when we feel beaten down and broken, but think of each day as a rebirth in which all kinds of good things and opportunities will present themselves. Have faith in you!

Two years ago Howard had severe heartburn. After two EKGs showed no indication of a heart attack, a troponin-level test showed that he was, indeed, having a heart attack. We remembered seeing Bill Clinton on David Letterman talking about his prevent-and-reverse-heart-disease diet. Googling that led us to Dr. Caldwell Esselstyn, and that in turn led us to attend the Engine 2 Seven-Day Rescue Immersion in Sedona, Arizona. Since then we have both lost weight, our blood pressure and cholesterol levels are excellent, and our energy is that of people fifteen years younger.

—Kerry Moskowitz, age 65, international student program coordinator; and Howard Moskowitz, age 58, construction business owner

Exercise Prevents Muscle Loss

It's an unfortunate truth: As you age, your muscles decay. It's a process called sarcopenia, and it begins right around your thirtieth birthday. After the big 3-0, people who are inactive can lose as much as 8 percent of their muscle mass per decade. Even if you are active, it gets harder and harder to retain that mass. As an athlete in my fifties, believe me, I know how unfair it is.

But, luckily, there is a treatment for sarcopenia. Nope, it doesn't come in a pill or a shake—it's good old-fashioned exercise! I look at my mother and father as shining examples of people who live the plant- and exercise-strong lifestyle to the max and have managed to keep the aging process at bay. Not only do they eat a whole-food, plant-based diet, they regularly engage in physical activity. My mother, Ann, is eighty-one and runs for an hour five days a week. The other two days she attends an hour-long yoga class. When the harsh Ohio winter settles in, Ann trades her running shoes for cross-country skis and glides across a nearby golf course. When not running or skiing, she is keeping two gardens, swimming, and playing tennis. She's a machine!

My father is no slouch either. Essy, as we call him, is eighty-three and heads out for an hour-long bike ride every day of the year unless the weather is bad, in which case he hops on his stationary bike. To combat sarcopenia, Essy lifts weights at least three days a week, stretches every morning, and swims whenever possible. Neither Ann nor Essy are on any medications, and they are still flying all over the world delivering lectures on the benefits of a whole food, plant-based diet.

I heard a story recently about a man named Charles Eugster, a ninety-seven-year-old retired dentist from England. Once a top rower, he found his strength diminishing as he aged. But Charles wasn't ready to go down without a fight. At the age of eighty-seven, he joined a bodybuilding club and hired a former Mr. Universe to whip him into shape. Fast-forward a decade, and Charles is now competing in the World Masters Athletics Championship. In fact, in 2015 Charles broke the world record for the 200-meter sprint in his age division by more than two seconds!

Treating Sore Muscles with Plants

As you age, nothing is better than resistance exercises to preserve your muscles. Unfortunately, sore muscles are a fact of life for people who lift weights or run hard. Soreness isn't all bad, of course—it indicates your muscles are getting stronger! But wouldn't it be nice to have a plant-strong remedy to help them bounce back faster?

You're in luck! I came across this awesome study in the *British Journal of Sports Medicine* recently that reveals the muscle-soothing power of cherries. The researchers found that male college athletes who consume cherries can reduce the strength loss associated with excessive bicep curls from 22 percent to just 4 percent. In another study, researchers out of the Oregon Health and Science University concluded that cherries "can minimize post-run muscle pain."

It turns out cherries aren't the only muscle-soothing plant around. Researchers out of Spain determined that two cups of watermelon can "reduce the recovery heart rate and muscle soreness" twenty-four hours after exercising.

> There's nothing wrong with a little soreness now and then, but why not eat some delicious fruit so you can get off the couch and head back to the gym!

I sure do love exercise!

When discussing plant-based eating, I often cede authority to nutrition experts such as my father and other plant-based luminaries like T. Colin Campbell and Neal Barnard. Their research is featured prominently in all my books, and they are probably the most knowledgeable people on the planet when it comes to preventing and reversing chronic disease through diet.

But boy, do I know exercise. I've been doing it regularly since I was an eight-year-old swimmer with the Lake Erie Silver Dolphins club in Cleveland, Ohio. Daily exercise has been a part of my existence for the past forty-five years. I've fallen in love with feeling at one with my body when I'm slicing through water during a swim, climbing a rock-strewn path on my mountain bike, bounding down the road on a run, or breathing mindfully during yoga. I love challenging, pushing, and developing my body. I love the pure joy that only exercise can give. Exercise is poetry in literal motion. It's pure beauty.

I realize that not everyone shares this love. That's totally fine! I don't expect you to enter the Ironman World Championship in Kona, Hawaii, after seven days. I don't expect you to do anything that doesn't feel good or doesn't make sense in your busy workaday life. But I do want you to engage in *some* sort of activity every day, even if it's only for five to ten minutes. Every last bit helps.

Exercise physiologist Timothy Church, who has studied exercise extensively, has this to say: "The greatest health benefit from exercise comes from getting up off the couch. Everything after that is incremental." According to the CDC, 80 percent of people in this country don't exercise on a regular basis. Perhaps this is because people associate exercise with athletic training. Since you're not reporting to spring training with the Texas Rangers, the thinking might go, maybe that morning jog isn't really necessary. But there is a big difference between exercising for sports performance and exercising for health. I want you to exercise for health.

I don't care what type of exercise you do as long as you just do it! I could give you a whole litany of amazing exercises, but instead I want to give you one exercise to do every day this week—one that doesn't require getting into your car, buying a gym membership, or wearing a special set of clothes. It's an exercise that almost everyone can do, with health benefits that include reducing your risk of heart disease, diabetes, obesity, high blood pressure, depression, and many other chronic ailments. You can do this exercise alone, with a friend, or with a group. You can go slow or fast. You can do this during the dog days of summer or the doldrums of winter.

And that one exercise is...drumroll...walking! Get out for a walk. Throw on some shoes, step out the door, and walk for ten, fifteen, thirty, or forty-five minutes.

Did you know that regular walking can help ward off the common cold and even the flu? One study out of Appalachian State University that followed 1,000 men and women found that walking briskly for thirty to forty-five minutes daily can increase the amount of immune cells circulating in the body. Moreover, the participants who walked the most—at least twenty minutes per day, five days a week—took 43 percent fewer sick days compared to individuals who exercised just once a week or less. So make walking a daily habit and don't look back!

Now, for those of you who want two more simple and effective exercises to complement your walking, here's what I want you to do:

> **Body-Weight Air Squats:** Do them anywhere, anytime. Standing in front of a chair, bench, or Swiss ball with your feet shoulder width apart, pretend you are going to sit down, lowering your bottom until it barely touches the surface. Then rise back up to the standing position. Form is important. Sit back into the squat with your heels, not your toes. Using good form, do 15 to 20 reps, and go down only as far as feels comfortable. Do two sets every day. Let them be the first thing on your mind when you get up and the last thing on your mind before you go to bed. Even better, perform them during work breaks and get your coworkers to join you!

Planks: This core exercise works the abs, the pelvic floor, the hips, and the stabilizing muscles of the back. Get ready for a sweet burn and, perhaps, to shake like a leaf. Remember to engage your abs and extend out through your head and through your feet. I challenge you to work up to five minutes of this exercise—and if you can, you are an Engine 2 workout animal!

To do the plank pose, lie facedown and place your toes and elbows on the ground. Then push up so your back is perfectly straight. Do these with your forearms on the ground (beginners, keep your knees on the ground as well). Hold for ten seconds and then take a ten-second break. Repeat five times. You're done in 1 minute and 30 seconds. Yes!

We all need to move. That's what our bodies are built to do. Find that missing joy that resides within all of us. In tandem with eating strong food, exercise will propel your health and happiness to new levels!

Conclusion

Congratulations! You've just digested seven lifesaving nuggets to rescue your life! This information may contradict much of what you read and hear in the media today. It takes a very special person to question the status quo—and that's you! By reading this book and embracing the Seven-Day Rescue, you have decided that you will not settle for mediocrity. You are ready to bust free from the chains that have kept you down and from the unhealthy relationships you have built up over a lifetime with food. You are ready to avoid a life of medications and constant doctor visits. You are ready to take charge of your health and master your own destiny.

For some of you, these seven days will be easy as plant-based pie. Others may struggle a little. But please know that it will be worth every step! At our seven-day retreats a few people do become unsettled. For example, one woman felt like we were telling her that the sky was green and the grass was blue. She couldn't get her brain wrapped around the seven major rescues that you've just read about. She was wrestling with how she was going to explain all of this new information on nutrition to her overweight and type 2 diabetic brothers, sisters, and parents. She could already hear their voices in her head: *You must eat meat for protein!*; *You need dairy for calcium!*; *Olive oil is heart-healthy!* It was all too much for her—that is, until the seven days were over and not only did she feel great, she couldn't wait to talk to her relatives!

This will happen to you, too. No matter what the doubters say when you start, when you finish, all healthy, slim, and happy, the questions you'll start hearing will include "Can you help me do this too?"; "When can I start?"; "How did you do it?"; "You did all that in how many days?"

So get revved up and start your journey! This is your opportunity to dazzle your insides, lose weight, and blow your doctor's mind! Head over to your doctor's office or the local drugstore and take a before selfie of your insides by getting a lipid panel of your total cholesterol, LDL cholesterol, HDL cholesterol, triglycerides, and a fasting blood sugar. Take a hard look at these numbers because this is the current you. Own it.

Now, commit to the Seven-Day Rescue. At the end of the week take an after selfie of your insides. You own this, too. Bring these new beautiful numbers to your doctor. She may well be at a loss for words. She may not even know that these kinds of results are possible in one week. So help your doctor out! Tell her what you did and why she should recommend it to all her patients!

The power of plant-strong food to protect, heal, and reverse disease has never been as timely as it is right now. Not next month, not next year— now! Now is the time to jump in and tackle the Seven-Day Rescue with all the gusto and heart you have.

The good news is: You can have it all! You can have insanely radical, radiant health and incredibly delicious food all at the same time. Now is the time for you to take the reins. Now is the time for you to take control. A healthy future lies in front of you, and all it takes is this one week to plant the seeds that will bear fruit for a lifetime. To learn more about the research cited in this book, please visit SevenDayRescue.com/Science.

PART II

8

The Seven-Day Rescue Plan

Let this week be a week for the ages. A week that will go down in your personal history book as the most life-changing, life-affirming seven days you've ever experienced. And it all starts here—with the food. This part of the Seven-Day Rescue is where we distill everything from the previous seven chapters into one week's worth of food and focus on creating habits that will have you eating strong, powerful food not just for one week but, I sincerely hope, for many years afterward.

Whom did I ask to help me with the recipes in this section of the Seven-Day Rescue? My sister Jane! There is no one I trust more in the kitchen. Jane is bursting with energy, ideas, creativity, and terrific recipes! She also brings a passionate perspective to the kitchen as a mom, a nurse, and a former Division I college athlete. She has helped me provide easy, step-by-step accessibility to the Seven-Day Rescue, just as she did in the recipe section of my last book, *Plant-Strong*. Jane also coauthored *The Prevent and Reverse Heart Disease Cookbook* with our mom, Ann.

Most recently, Jane's expertise was called upon when the Cleveland Clinic conducted a study on the effects of a plant-based diet on pediatric obesity and high cholesterol. Jane worked with doctors and researchers to provide the curriculum, recipes, cooking demonstrations, and other materials for the monthlong endeavor. The landmark results were published in the *Journal of Pediatrics* in February 2015.

Welcome to Rip and Jane's Rescue Kitchen for seven wonderful days!

The concept of giving up cheese, ice cream, butter, and fish was on my mind constantly! Luckily my mom also did the challenge with me. But by the third day my mind had shifted to finding new and exciting recipes to make plant-strong!

The rest of the week was filled with LOTS of food. In the end the number I was most interested in was not my weight, which did improve, but my blood pressure—it went from 178/90 to 148/88, which was an improvement that previously took me six months to obtain through regular dieting (and then went right back up when I could no longer stay on a heavily restricted diet). For me it's important to feel some pleasure from food; my mind just can't see it as fuel alone, so trying new recipes was critical for me, and I found a ton that were wonderful!

—Lynn Westfall, age 33,
IT procurement administrator

OVERVIEW

During these next seven days, your plate will be filled with nothing but healing, strong foods. This means that you will:

1. Consume no meat. Don't even think about beef, turkey, chicken, pork, fish, venison, or shellfish. Got the picture? You will eat nothing that had a mother, nothing that had a face, nothing that ever pooped.

2. Consume no dairy products or eggs. In other words, nothing that comes from a cow, goat, or any other animal. Not in any form: no milk, butter, cheese, cream, ice cream, cream cheese, sour cream, cottage cheese, ricotta cheese, Parmesan cheese, ghee, or anything containing eggs—no yolks and no whites.

3. Use no added oil. Oil, no matter what type, is 100 percent fat. All the oils and essential fat we need exist in the proper proportions in whole foods. There is no need to extract them from the olive, corn, coconut, sunflower, or any other whole plants. Consuming food in its whole intact form is the best way to get the proper amount of essential fats we need. This also means no cooking spray—it is possible to cook without oil in the pan. And this means yes to nonstick pans and parchment paper, your new best friends for roasting and baking.

4. Go easy on the nuts and avocados. Nuts are little inflammatory fat bombs that are similar to potato chips (you can't eat just one). During the next seven days, the only nuts that will be entering your mouth are walnuts. Walnuts have an excellent omega-3 to omega-6 ratio, unlike almost every other nut. The catch is, we want your daily walnut consumption to be one small handful, the equivalent of 200 calories. More is not better. Avocados are to be consumed in small amounts and eliminated entirely if you have heart disease, diabetes, or are trying to lose weight. This has to do with their high fat content and how easy it is to overeat guacamole and avocados. Some recipes call for one whole avocado, but this is meant to be split over four servings. Again, because walnuts are so calorie-dense and avocados are so high in fat, we need to eat them sparingly, or not at all.

5. Eat greens at every meal. Greens at lunch and dinner are familiar to most of us. But what about breakfast? Sticking a little spinach into your Savory Spinach Steel-Cut Oats (page 204) is amazing. Soon greens will taste delicious and even feel welcome at each meal. At our weeklong Rescues, we always serve green leafy vegetables at breakfast, lunch, and dinner. At first some participants say, "You gotta be kidding me!" but by the end of the week, their plates are heaped with kale, collards, spinach, broccoli, or bok choy! Check out the "Dressings, Hummus, Toppings, and Sides" section (page 257) to find some great sauces for your daily greens. Our goal is to get three to six servings of greens a day.

6. Steer clear of animal protein. By doing so, you will steer clear of disease! According to our leading nutritional researchers, around 6–10 percent of your diet should be made up of protein. Any percentage higher than 10 percent is associated with an increase of disease. So stop obsessing about protein. It's a waste of your time, energy, and money.

7. Consume minimal salt. *Minimal* means "little to none." There are many other ways to spice up your food: vinegar, balsamic glaze, spices, herbs, lemon juice and zest, lime juice and zest, other citrus fruit juices and zest. We also like low-sodium tamari sauce, which happens to be gluten-free, but be mindful, because even the low-sodium variety still is packed with sodium. Read labels and keep the milligrams of sodium per serving equal to or less than the number of calories per serving (see chapter 6). Condiments such as ketchup, mustard, hummus, tamari, and pasta sauce can have as much as a 5:1 ratio of milligrams of sodium to calories per serving.

8. Consume minimal sugar. Again, *minimal* means "little to none." We prefer 100 percent pure maple syrup in recipes, and very occasionally we may choose a product like barbecue sauce or ketchup that contains sugar. Be very careful of the added sugar in packaged and canned products. You will find during the seven days how much you enjoy naturally sweet whole foods such as oats, carrots, beets, and sweet potatoes! Refer to chapter 6 for our Rescue guidelines regarding added sugars.

9. Consume 100 percent whole grains. This week our focus is going to be on whole grains for all the reasons discussed in chapter 2. Oats are featured in almost all our breakfasts, because their health benefits are magical. Oats are dose-responsive—in other words, the more you eat, the more good they do! Oats help lower cholesterol, lower blood sugar, and decrease arterial inflammation. Eat them each day in their simplest forms: steel-cut oats or old-fashioned oats. Steer away from packets of salted and sweetened oatmeal and quick oats. What's one of the many things that make whole grains so great? Fiber. Fiber fills you up and it keeps your bowels moving and supple. Different whole grains have unique flavors and textures, all of which rescue your health. Try them all and discover which ones you love.

10.   Drink lots of water. Tap, sparkling, flat, warm, cold, icy, with a squeeze of lemon, lime, or other citrus fruit, or steeped herbal tea. No sodas, smoothies, or juices this week. Over your lifetime, you will save thousands of calories and thousands of dollars if you stick with water.

SEVEN DAYS OF MEALS

This week you will enjoy twenty-one meals that are plant-strong and filled with vitality; twenty-one powerful meals that will nurture you as you take a deep dive to where nutrition really lives. Get ready to have it your way as we provide you with options that suit your personality and your palate. Over the course of our seven-day pilot studies, the participants have included people who love cooking, people who hate cooking, people who buy all their meals, and people who prefer to eat the same foods every day. In other words, these seven days will work for anyone, everyone, and, most important, you!

The core of your meals this week will be customized Rescue Bowls that you'll make following our simple Rescue Bowl guidelines. This casual style was a huge hit in our pilot studies. What's not to like when something is fast, easy, and personalized? Bowls totally rock whether they're for breakfast, lunch, or dinner! After all, a bowl can be filled anytime, anywhere with any plant-strong foods. Whereas once people had cereal for breakfast, a sandwich for lunch, and a heavy entrée for dinner, today it's not unusual to find people selecting a heaping bowl of salad greens for breakfast, savory bowls of noodles for lunch, and cereal bowls for dinner. This is your chance to eat what you want, when you want!

In case you start feeling the urge to break from your bowls for a meal or two, you'll also have your pick of Rescue Flats. A flat is what we call an open-faced sandwich (i.e., just one slice of bread with a heaping helping of wonderful strong foods on top). You'll find many mouthwatering recipes for these popular open-faced sandwiches, wraps, and pizzas in the Lunch section.

In addition to bowls and flats, you'll have your pick of mounds of delicious recipes that will light up your breakfast, lunch, and dinner. And because we don't want to leave any stone unturned, we'll be showing you more than forty super-simple "no-recipe recipe" combinations that you can whip up in a jiff (see pages 254–256).

The following is an example of how you might want to structure your meals for the week:

Seven-Day Rescue	Breakfast	Lunch	Dinner
Day 1	Easy Blueberry Oatmeal	Hummus and Avocado Flat	Brown Rice Bowl
Day 2	Banana Steel-Cut Oats	Split Pea Potato Soup	Southwestern Potato Bowl
Day 3	Big Bowl Mix	All-Day Kale Salad	Sweet Potato Bowl
Day 4	Purple Oatmeal	Red Pepper Smile Flat	Red Quinoa Bowl
Day 5	Peachy Keen Steel-Cut Oats	Bellissima Pasta Salad	Mighty Green Pasta Bowl
Day 6	Cinnamon Stick Oatmeal	Miso Barley Soup	Quinoa Cali Rolls
Day 7	Savory Spinach Steel-Cut Oats	Black Bean and Sprouts Flat	Sloppy Joe Tostados

Remember, we don't care what you eat or how you eat it. Follow the suggestions in the grid, or come up with your own week of plant-strong meals. Whatever works best for you!

Also, if you want to plan your meals ahead of time, consider batch cooking—many Engine 2 fans love to cook all their food in one weekend so they don't have to spend time on their meals the rest of the week.

But hey, if you don't feel like planning, then skip right ahead to the recipes on pages 194–268!

BATCH COOKING: COOK NOW, EAT LATER!

If you fail to prepare, you are preparing to fail.
—Attributed to Benjamin Franklin

For many, the downfall of healthy eating is the failure to plan ahead. Planning helps prevent the pitfall of impulsive, caught-in-the-moment, mindless, fill-the-tank-now gorging. If you wait until you are running on empty and growling with hunger, impulsive eating will take over.

Fear not. Batch cooking is here to prevent those pitfalls. Batch cooking simply means the preparation of a mega-amount of food ahead of time—perhaps on a Sunday evening, for example—so that you can breeze through the rest of the week without having to cook. It might look something like this: during a football game or an episode of *Masterpiece Theatre*, bake a tray of sweet potatoes and white potatoes, while also making a pot of rice or quinoa in the rice cooker and a pot of oatmeal on the stovetop.

While all is cooking, toss a mix of dry cereals together, such as the Big Bowl Mix (page 200). After an hour or less of cooking, this batch of food is done! Wrap, seal, or store everything to be used in meals for the week ahead (it's definitely worth it to invest in some good food storage containers). You are ready for oatmeal-based or dry cereal breakfast bowls. You are ready for a hearty salad bowl or to build your own bowl. Day by day, you will use everything you prepared in various ways: rice, quinoa, polenta, and sweet potatoes or potatoes (diced, cubed, smashed, or whole), reheated then covered with veggies, beans, salsa, and spices or hot sauce. Delicious!

Another option for saving time are what we call "batch recipes." This refers to doubling or tripling a recipe to be wrapped, sealed, and stored in the fridge or frozen for the week. This method is great for soups, stews, burritos, quesadillas, and burgers. You can prepare these recipes yourself, or you can take a more communal approach. Have five friends come over to cook one recipe times five. At the end of your batch cooking hangout, you will each be stocked with five recipes for the week!

Also, note that many frozen or vacuum-packed grains are available and are compliant with our guidelines. The Engine 2 product line has numerous options of frozen grains, prepared hummus, wraps, veggie burgers, burger buns, pizza crusts, and crispbreads as well. And, you can buy plain frozen brown rice and quinoa in many stores.

Whether cooking from scratch or creating heat-and-go meals, the approach that will work best for you is the one that allows you to eat strong foods. Use the simple and quick combo of fresh foods like apples, bananas, prewashed salad greens and presliced veggies (available in the produce section), or frozen veggies, on top of or mixed in with your precooked oats, potatoes, and grains (frozen or precooked). Then top everything off with salsa, hot sauce, or one of our Rescue dressings.

Batch Cooking Grocery List

When drawing up a shopping list for the week, be sure to start by including your preferred foods as well as the ingredients you'll need to try a handful of the recipes we have provided. This will ensure that you have a winning week!

To create your grocery list, use the grid of E2 recipes from page 184, or make your own grid by thinking *7, 7, 7*:

- 7 breakfasts
- 7 lunches
- 7 dinners

It will look something like this:

- 7 breakfasts: oatmeal, dry cereals, fresh fruits, frozen blueberries, frozen mangoes, almond milk, spinach
- 7 lunches: whole wheat pita bread, Ezekiel bread, hummus, tomatoes, cucumbers, green onions, cilantro, balsamic glaze, heads of romaine lettuce
- 7 dinners: sweet potatoes, brown rice, whole wheat pasta, canned beans, kale, cherry tomatoes, garlic, mushrooms, frozen corn, broccoli, cumin, spices, lemons, and limes
- Items like whole fruit and extra vegetables and hummus for snacks

Tips: The amount of each item depends on the number of people in your household. Check what condiments and spices you have at home before you head to the store.

Seven Batch Cooking Tips:

1. Purchase items like parchment paper and freezer-friendly food storage containers before you batch cook. If you can, store foods in portion-size containers. Freeze items like soups, burritos, burgers, brown rice, and beans. They are all easy to heat up again later.
2. Spend fifteen minutes plotting out a menu for the week. It will pay off in spades! See the example grid of E2 recipes for the week on page 184.
3. On the day of batch cooking, have a plan. Preheat your oven and start with the things that will take the longest to cook (generally potatoes).
4. Make A LOT of potatoes! Sweet, red, yellow, whatever you like. Potatoes are a great staple to have in your house for meals or snacks.
5. Chop up fruits and vegetables and put them in storage containers so that you always have fresh produce ready to go without prep time.
6. Make a few plant-strong dressings for the week.
7. Get the family involved!

Rescue Batch Cooking Simple Shopping List

Use the following list as a guideline. Add items you love, like mango or oregano, and skip those you don't love.

> **VEGGIES:** Pick your favorite items here. What do you like in a salad? Look for steam-in-the-bag potatoes to save time. Steam-in-the-bag vegetables are great time-savers as well.

Beets
Bell peppers
Broccoli
Canned tomatoes
Carrots
Celery
Collard greens
Engine 2 Pasta Sauce
Frozen veggies
Green onions
Kale
Salad greens
Spinach
Tomatoes
Whole onions
Zucchini

FRUIT: Pick your favorite items here. Do you like some fruit in your salad? What fruit do you like to snack on? If frozen, the products should be single ingredient items, no salt or sugar added.

Apples
Applesauce
Bananas
Berries
Grapes
Kiwis
Lemons
Limes
Mandarin oranges
Nectarines
Oranges
Peaches

GRAINS: Buy brown rice, black rice, red rice, or any color of quinoa in bulk to save money. To save time, look for brown rice, quinoa, farro, or other grains in freezer or shelf-stable containers. Always read labels, and remember, no oil, dairy, or eggs in breads. Look for Engine 2 brand whole-grain pizza crusts, cereals, crispbread crackers, tortillas, grain blends, and burger buns at Whole Foods Market.

100 percent oil-free whole-grain bread
100 percent oil-free whole-grain pizza crust
100 percent oil-free whole-grain pizza tortillas
100 percent whole-grain pasta
Brown rice
Corn tortillas
Grape-Nuts or Ezekiel 4:9 Cereal
Old-fashioned oats
Polenta
Potatoes—any variety
Quinoa
Shredded wheat
Sweet potatoes
Uncle Sam Cereal

BEANS/LEGUMES: Pick your favorite beans. Save time: Buy cans (no salt added). Save money: Buy dried beans and cook in bulk. Dry lentils are quick and cheap, especially red lentils.

Adzuki beans
Black beans
Black-eyed peas
Butter beans
Cannellini beans
Chickpeas
Fat-free vegetarian refried beans
Kidney beans
Lentils
Oil-free hummus
Pinto beans

SPICES, ETC.: Look for salt-free blends in the spice section of your grocery store. A smoky mesquite blend, a garlic blend, a curry blend, and a spicy fiesta blend make cooking easy. Look in the bulk section for nutritional yeast. See what you already have in your cupboard before heading to the store.

Black pepper
Chia seed
Chili powder
Cinnamon
Cumin
Curry powder
Flax meal
Nutritional yeast
Oregano
Rosemary
Salt-free seasoning blends
Thyme
Your favorite spices

CONDIMENTS: These are items we use sparingly. Shoot for low-sodium products and no high-fructose corn syrup. Pick items that you enjoy, but follow the "No oil" rule. Get real, 100 percent pure maple syrup. What do you already have in your cupboard?

Balsamic vinegar
Barbecue sauce
Hot sauce
Ketchup
Low-sodium tamari
Maple syrup
Mustard
Salsa
Sriracha hot sauce, or your own favorite hot sauce
Unsweetened almond milk
Unsweetened oat milk

Jill, on Prepping the Night Before

I have never been a morning person, so over the years I've had to learn how to make sure my mornings run as smoothly as possible. When I was a teacher, and then an administrator, I used to prepare all my meeting or lesson materials the night before, setting every item out just the way it needed to be in order to start off the day. I knew I would not do anything but be a warm body the next morning, so I had to set everything up exactly how I wanted it!

The same thing goes for preparing breakfasts for my kids in the morning. I actually got the idea from reading Beverly Cleary's *Ramona the Pest* with our kids. Ramona's mom, Mrs. Quimby, was setting the table for breakfast when Ramona was going to bed. Of course! What a great idea. So that's what I do now. If we're having oatmeal, the night before I measure 2 cups of water into a pot and cover it on the stove. Next to it, I keep the one-cup measure of oatmeal. I set out a cutting board and knife for the fruit I'm going to serve in the morning. I set out bowls and spoons at the kids' places. If we're having Rip's granola or Big Bowl, I'll take it out of the pantry and set it on the table.

It's so much easier for me to walk into our kitchen with a set table and food in the initial stages of preparation than an empty kitchen, especially with my superfoggy brain, a one-year-old who won't let me put her down until she has some food on her plate, a six-year-old who wants to draw instead of putting on her socks and shoes, and an eight-year-old who would rather throw his football against the wall all morning than eat.

Rip and Jill on Batch Cooking

When our household takes on a Seven-Day Rescue, we make sure to have plenty of food containers of varying sizes and parchment paper. On Sunday, our batch cooking day, we bake six large sweet potatoes and a dozen Yukon Gold potatoes. We boil six large beets and make a huge pot of oatmeal and six cups of brown rice. We have our triple-washed greens in the big visible container, and our favorite, black beans, drained and rinsed in a sealed container in the fridge. These foods provide the foundation for all of our bowls in no time. And Jill has at her beck and call three naturally sweet foods: sweet potatoes, beets, and oats, which never fail to curb her sweet tooth that always seems to rear its ugly head either midafternoon or right before bed.

Jane and Brian on Batch Cooking

My husband and I have three teenage athletes in our house, so our batch cooking never ends! On Sunday we make as much brown rice as our rice cooker can hold! This will be used during the week for black beans and Brown Rice Bowls, Launcher Quesadillas, Gallo Pinto Salad, and Quinoa Cali Rolls as the week goes on. We cook a tray of sweet potatoes and a sack of Yukon Gold potatoes, which all get used in a variety of ways during the week as well: Sweet Potato Bowls, Southwestern Potato Bowls, various soups, and potato wedges (sliced, spiced, and reheated on a parchment-lined tray!). Also, we have heaps of beans in Tupperware, stacks of tortillas (in corn, rice, and whole-grain varieties), jars of plant-strong dressings, and bags of spring greens, washed and at the ready.

Midweek we prepare a four-cup pot of red quinoa. This is used as a foundation in bowls, as a way to power up salads, or mixed in with soups. We have broccoli every night, so each week we buy a brimming bag of broccoli crowns that can be broken by hand and set to steaming in a flash.

Also, we find that if we slice up fruit such as oranges, watermelon, cantaloupe, strawberries, and grapefruit, the kids gobble it up. One night our son ate twenty-seven orange slices! If we don't slice it up, it tends to sit untouched.

A LAST WORD

Approach this week well-armed with everything you've read in this book. For some of you these seven days may seem a little difficult, while others will immediately fall in love with their new plant-based foods. For all of you: Hang in there for seven days and don't let go! Eat as many Rescue Bowls as you want. Try some Rescue Flats. Test your cooking skills in the kitchen with the Rescue recipes. Make time one afternoon or evening and batch cook for the week.

Above all, find what resonates best with your palate and your lifestyle and dig in with every fiber of your being. Make this a week you will never forget. You deserve to eat well, live well, feel well, and achieve greatness. By the end of the seven days, you'll be fluent in shopping for, cooking, and eating plant-strong foods that will fuel your strength for a happy and healthier you!

9

Seven-Day Rescue Recipes

BREAKFAST

Rescue Breakfast Bowls

Wow yourself with the size of your big cereal bowl. Pile it so high that you are still eating it in the carpool line at the preschool drop-off, on the train to work, in the midmorning meeting at the office, or on the way to your 10:00 a.m. yoga class! Building a breakfast bowl is as easy as 1-2-3. You've done it thousands of times. Now you can do it with nutritious gusto! We've had more people tell us that the big bowl first thing in the morning was the linchpin to their success and laid the foundation for the day.

Of course, if you want to end your day with a great big cereal bowl, that's terrific. These bowls are easy ways to make plant-strong meals anytime at all.

ENGINE 2 RESCUE

BREAKFAST BOWL

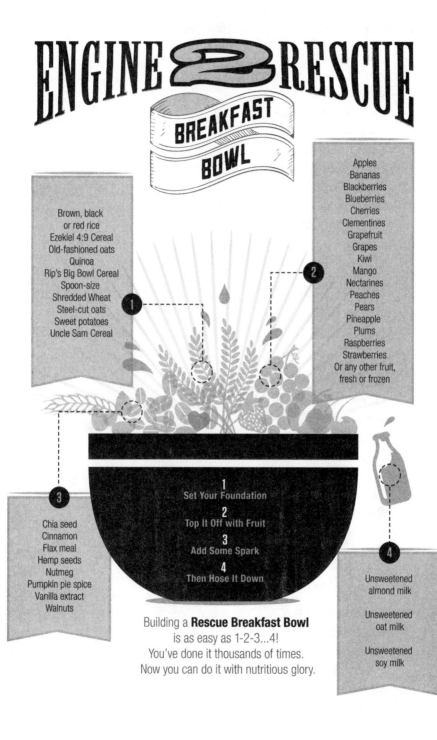

1
Brown, black
or red rice
Ezekiel 4:9 Cereal
Old-fashioned oats
Quinoa
Rip's Big Bowl Cereal
Spoon-size
Shredded Wheat
Steel-cut oats
Sweet potatoes
Uncle Sam Cereal

2
Apples
Bananas
Blackberries
Blueberries
Cherries
Clementines
Grapefruit
Grapes
Kiwi
Mango
Nectarines
Peaches
Pears
Pineapple
Plums
Raspberries
Strawberries
Or any other fruit,
fresh or frozen

3
Chia seed
Cinnamon
Flax meal
Hemp seeds
Nutmeg
Pumpkin pie spice
Vanilla extract
Walnuts

4
Unsweetened
almond milk

Unsweetened
oat milk

Unsweetened
soy milk

1
Set Your Foundation

2
Top It Off with Fruit

3
Add Some Spark

4
Then Hose It Down

Building a **Rescue Breakfast Bowl**
is as easy as 1-2-3...4!
You've done it thousands of times.
Now you can do it with nutritious glory.

Building Your Rescue Breakfast Bowls

SET YOUR FOUNDATION . . .

Brown, black, or red rice

Ezekiel 4:9 Cereal

Old-fashioned oats

Quinoa

Rip's Big Bowl Cereal

Spoon-size shredded wheat

Steel-cut oats

Sweet potatoes

Uncle Sam Cereal

THEN TOP IT OFF WITH FRUIT . . .

Apples

Bananas

Blackberries

Blueberries

Cherries

Clementines

Grapefruit

Grapes

Kiwi

Mango

Nectarines

Peaches

Pears

Pineapple

Plums

Raspberries

Strawberries

Or any other fruit you can think of—fresh or frozen

ADD SOME SPARK . . .

Chia seed

Cinnamon

Flax meal

Hemp seeds

Nutmeg

Pumpkin pie spice
Vanilla extract
Walnuts

THEN HOSE IT DOWN WITH ...
Unsweetened almond milk
Unsweetened oat milk
Unsweetened soy milk

Dig in and enjoy your cold-cereal breakfast bowl, or, if your oatmeal, quinoa, or sweet potato needs to be heated up, throw it in the microwave!

Rip's Favorite: In a big bowl, lay a foundation of raw old-fashioned oats or Rip's Big Bowl Cereal, top it with frozen mango chunks (thawed in the microwave for 45 seconds), a sliced banana, grapefruit slices, and a spark of chia seeds, then hose it down with oat milk or almond milk.

Here are ten cereal bowl recipes we can't get enough of!

Easy Blueberry Oatmeal

Just like it sounds. Easy prep, add blueberries, gobble it up. Prepare the oats raw or cooked!

Serves 2

INGREDIENTS:

2 cups water
1 cup old-fashioned oats
1 tablespoon chia seeds or ground
    flaxseed meal

1 banana, peeled and sliced
½ cup blueberries (fresh or frozen)

INSTRUCTIONS:

In a small pot over high heat, bring the water and oats to a boil. Reduce the heat to low and simmer for 2 to 3 minutes while stirring occasionally. When the oatmeal becomes the desired texture, remove the pot from the heat. Heap the cooked oatmeal into bowls, top with chia seeds, banana, and blueberries (thaw a bit first if using frozen berries). Serve and enjoy!

Banana Steel-Cut Oats

Steel-cut oats are named after the way they are processed. Large steel blades chop whole oat groats into two or three pieces. This process creates a chewier and coarser texture than rolled oats. This steel-cut recipe makes the kitchen smell like there's banana bread in the oven—the ultimate comfort food! And this warm, sweet, filling breakfast will put a banana-size smile on your face!

Serves 2

INGREDIENTS:

1 ripe spotted banana, smashed in its own skin
3 cups water
1 teaspoon vanilla
1 cup steel-cut oats
1 tablespoon chia seeds or ground flaxseed meal
¼ teaspoon cinnamon
⅛ teaspoon ground nutmeg
1 kiwi, peeled and sliced
¼ cup strawberries or berries of choice (fresh or frozen), sliced

INSTRUCTIONS:

In a small pot over medium heat, mix the smashed banana (no skin), water, and vanilla.

Add the steel-cut oats, bring to a boil, cover, and reduce the heat to a simmer. Stir occasionally so the oats don't stick to the bottom. Cook for 15 to 20 minutes, depending on how chewy you prefer your oats. If you like smoother oats, cook a few minutes longer. Add the chia seeds, cinnamon, and nutmeg and stir. Serve in bowls topped with kiwi and strawberries. These oats are surprisingly sweet alone.

Raw Old-Fashioned Strawberry Oats

Raw oats may seem a little odd at first, but they aren't really raw. They've already been steamed and rolled, and you'll come to appreciate and love them. Make this bowl the same way you made your bowl of Cap'n Crunch or Count Chocula as a kid: Fill up your bowl, pour on the nondairy milk, and go. If you are using frozen strawberries, thaw them first in the microwave, then slice before adding to the mix.

Serves 2

INGREDIENTS:

1 to 2 cups old-fashioned oats
Almond or oat milk, enough to
   fill the bowl to your liking
1 tablespoon chia seeds or
   ground flaxseed meal

1 kiwi, peeled and sliced
1 banana, peeled and sliced
½ cup strawberries (fresh or frozen),
   sliced

INSTRUCTIONS:

Place the raw oats in your bowl (as much has you like). Pour the almond milk over the oats (just like any other bowl of dry cereal). Some people prefer the milk to cover the top, and some like it just on the bottom. Use whatever amount you prefer. Top off with chia seeds, kiwi, banana, and strawberries. Hug your bowl, grab your spoon, and dig in!

Triple Berry Oatmeal

This is a year-round berry of a breakfast treat! We love berries because of the high-octane amounts of antioxidants and phytonutrients that are stuffed into their little juicy bodies. Blackberries, raspberries, blueberries, strawberries, or gooseberries! Fresh or frozen, juice up your body with a bunch of berries today!

Serves 2

INGREDIENTS:

1¾ to 2 cups water, depending on how thick (less water) or thin (more water) you prefer your oatmeal

1 cup old-fashioned oats

1 tablespoon chia seeds or ground flaxseed meal

½ cup blueberries (fresh or frozen)

½ cup raspberries (fresh or frozen)

½ cup strawberries (fresh or frozen), sliced

INSTRUCTIONS:

Place a small pot over high heat and bring the water to a boil. Add the oats, reduce the heat, and cook 2 to 5 minutes (depending on how chewy you like your oats) while stirring occasionally. Serve in 2 breakfast bowls, topped with chia seeds and heaped with blueberries, raspberries, and strawberries, or the berries of your choosing.

Big Bowl Mix

This recipe makes a full fire truckload of food! It will last a family of five for the week—or one breakfast-loving, midnight-snacking firefighter (Rip) for one week! This is the original mix that Rip used to eat, which inspired his Engine 2 Rip's Big Bowl cereals. For some people, dry cereal in the morning is all they need. A big bowl of this mix will keep you flying high until lunch. Again, this makes a ton of cereal, so if you are preparing it for just one person, cut the recipe in half for the week or by one quarter for two to three breakfasts.

INGREDIENTS FOR MIX:

1 (24-ounce) box Grape-Nuts Cereal

1 (42-ounce) container old-fashioned oats

1 (13-ounce) box Uncle Sam flake cereal

1 (18-ounce) box spoon-size shredded wheat

SERVE WITH:

Oat milk, almond milk, or soy milk

1 banana, sliced

½ cup blueberries or berries or fruit of choice

1 tablespoon chia seeds or ground flaxseed meal

INSTRUCTIONS:

In a large sealable container, combine equal parts of each cereal. Mix the dry cereals so they are equally dispersed. Fill your cereal bowl with a heaping helping of the dry mix and tightly seal the container. Add as much non-dairy milk to your bowl as you'd like, top with banana slices, blueberries, and chia seeds and start your day!

Overnight Applesauce Oats

These clever oats set you ahead for the week. Wake up, heat up a jar of your Overnight Applesauce Oats, and off you go each morning. The simple ingredients combine perfectly and store easily overnight (or all week) in the fridge. This recipe is a batch cooking favorite: it takes no time to make, and all six servings are stored in lidded mason jars or Tupperware containers ready for the taking.

Makes six 12-ounce servings

INGREDIENTS:

3 cups rolled oats
1 teaspoon cinnamon
1 teaspoon pumpkin spice

3 cups unsweetened applesauce
3 cups water

INSTRUCTIONS:

In a medium bowl, combine the oats, cinnamon, and pumpkin spice, then stir in the applesauce. Evenly distribute the oat mixture among 6 (12-ounce) jars with lids (like empty salsa jars) or other containers of equal size, and top each with ½ cup water. Place the lids on the jars or other containers and store in the refrigerator overnight. When ready to serve, heat the prepared oatmeal in the microwave for 1 minute or until warmed through—or enjoy it cold. This jarred breakfast lasts for 6 days, one jar per day. Perfect!

Purple Oatmeal

This breakfast wins on all fronts: the purple color appeals to little kids, teenagers dig the high drama of the color, and the antioxidants score big points with the adults.

Serves 2

INGREDIENTS:

2 cups water
½ cup steel-cut oats
1 cup frozen blueberries
1 teaspoon cinnamon

1 tablespoon chia seeds or ground flaxseed meal
½ cup raspberries or berries of choice (fresh or frozen)

INSTRUCTIONS:

Place the water in a small saucepan over high heat and bring to a boil.

Add the oats, lower the heat to medium, and simmer for 10 to 15 minutes, stirring occasionally. When the oats begin to gel and swell, add the frozen blueberries and cinnamon and stir. Continue cooking for 5 to 10 minutes or until the mixture reaches the preferred consistency.

Pour into bowls and serve topped with chia seeds and raspberries just before eating.

Peachy Keen Steel-Cut Oats

Peachy keen—because peaches are sweet, delicate, and special— just like you! Do not forget frozen fruit, as this makes Peachy Keen oatmeal an easy year-round option!

Serves 2

INGREDIENTS:

3 cups water
1 cup steel-cut oats
1 tablespoon chia seeds or ground flaxseed meal

1 peach (fresh or frozen), sliced
½ cup raspberries (fresh or frozen)

INSTRUCTIONS:

In a small pot over high heat, bring the water to a boil and add the oats. Reduce the heat to low and allow the oats to simmer for 10 to 20 minutes (depending on how chewy you like your oats) while stirring occasionally. Cover with a lid before removing from the heat and let stand a few minutes.

Serve in 2 breakfast bowls topped with chia seeds, peach slices (allow to thaw first if using frozen), and raspberries.

Cinnamon Stick Oatmeal

The cinnamon stick is magical in this recipe. It gives the oats a low level of sweetness and a hue of cinnamon flavor that cannot be created with any other ingredient. Ask your grocer where you can find these wonderful sticks. Sometimes they are in the baking aisle; sometimes they are in the bulk section. Take the time to find them and light up your oatmeal!

Serves 2

INGREDIENTS:

2 cups water
1 cup old-fashioned oats
1 cinnamon stick
1 tablespoon chia seeds or ground
    flaxseed meal

1 banana, peeled and sliced
¼ cup blueberries (fresh or frozen)

INSTRUCTIONS:

In a small pot over high heat, combine the water, oats, and cinnamon stick. Bring to a boil, then turn the heat down to a simmer and cook for 5 more minutes, stirring occasionally.

Remove the cinnamon stick, pour the oatmeal into 2 bowls, and gobble this up topped with chia seeds, banana slices, and blueberries (allow to thaw first if using frozen berries).

My goal was for the Seven-Day Rescue to be a jump start to change relatively unhealthy eating habits, with a short-term goal of losing weight. I was surprised by how good the plant-based diet could taste. I was also surprised at how easy it was to put the meals together and how full I felt after each meal. Overall, I never felt like I was denying myself anything with regard to either taste or quantity.

—Don Hook, age 66, retired certified
financial planner

Savory Spinach Steel-Cut Oats

If you're not in the mood for a sweet breakfast, this is your ticket. This recipe has the perfect combo of oat-healthy benefits and savory deliciousness. Try it. Seriously. The nutritional yeast gives a wonderful creaminess. On a cold day, this warms you inside and out, and you get those great breakfast greens to boot.

Serves 2

INGREDIENTS:

¾ cup steel-cut oats
2½ cups water
3 tablespoons nutritional yeast
¼ teaspoon turmeric
¾ cup mushrooms, sliced (optional but delicious; we like shitake)

1½ teaspoons sriracha sauce or hot sauce of choice
3 cups packed fresh spinach
1 tablespoon chia seeds or ground flaxseed meal

INSTRUCTIONS:

In a small saucepan, combine the oats, water, nutritional yeast, turmeric, mushrooms, and sriracha sauce.

Bring the mixture to a boil, watching carefully and stirring to prevent burning.

When the mixture just comes to a boil, reduce the heat to maintain a simmer and cook, stirring occasionally, for 10 to 12 minutes, until the water has been absorbed and the oats are creamy. Stir in the spinach and continue to cook until the spinach is tender.

Pour into bowls, sprinkle with chia seeds, and taste the savory goodness.

Rescue Family Breakfasts

Oat Pancakes

We eat these by the stack—a mile high! The key to this recipe is to start with old-fashioned oats. At first we tried oat flour, but it just didn't do the trick. For the best results, begin with regular old-fashioned oats and grind them into a flour with a high-speed blender or food processor.

Makes eight 4-inch pancakes

INGREDIENTS:

1½ cups old-fashioned oats
½ teaspoon baking soda
1 teaspoon baking powder
Pinch of salt (optional)
½ teaspoon cinnamon
Pinch of ground nutmeg
Pinch of ground cloves
2 teaspoons vanilla extract

¼ cup unsweetened applesauce, plus more for serving, if desired
Zest and juice of 1 orange
½ brown banana, smashed
1 cup almond milk
Quick Blueberry Topping (page 262)
Fresh fruit, for serving

INSTRUCTIONS:

Place the oats, baking soda, baking powder, salt (if using), cinnamon, nutmeg, and cloves in a high-speed blender and pulse until a coarse flour mixture is formed.

Pour the mixture into a medium bowl and add the vanilla, applesauce, orange zest and juice, banana, and almond milk. Stir well. Add more almond milk if the batter is too thick.

Heat a nonstick skillet over medium heat. Pour a large spoonful of batter into the hot skillet and wait for bubbles to form on the surface. Using a nonmetal spatula, flip the pancake over. Cook for another minute or until the underside is golden brown. Serve with blueberry topping and fresh fruit, or just unsweetened applesauce.

I went through the recipes and picked my favorites. I figured out how many servings I would get from each recipe and designed a weeklong meal plan. I then made a grocery list from this. Once I made the soup, sloppy joes, and breakfast patties, the week's meals and snacks became easier. I thought the recipes were very easy— especially the oat waffles! Overall, the meals were easy to follow, and I can't wait to try more of these recipes!

—Julie Wise, age 26, MS, RDN, LD

Oat Waffles

These waffles rule: kids love them, neighbors love them, dogs love them! Make the whole batch over the weekend, freeze extras, and throw two in the toaster for a midweek breakfast on the go— that is, if the kids, neighbors, dogs, or you haven't eaten them all!

Makes 6 square waffles

INGREDIENTS:

2½ cups old-fashioned oats
¼ cup flaxseed meal
Zest of 1 lemon
½ teaspoon cinnamon
1 medium banana, smashed

1½ cups almond milk
Quick Blueberry Topping
(page 262)
Fresh fruit, for serving (optional)

INSTRUCTIONS:

Preheat a nonstick waffle iron.

In a food processor or a high-speed blender, combine the oats, flaxseed meal, lemon zest, and cinnamon. Blend until the mixture reaches a flour-like texture.

To a medium bowl, add the oat mixture, the smashed banana, and the almond milk. Mix thoroughly with a fork (the batter will be fairly thick).

Portion the batter onto the preheated waffle iron and spread it around to all corners. Close the lid and cook per the waffle iron manufacturer's instructions. Gently remove the waffles when done. Make all the batter into waffles and save any leftovers for another day.

Serve with blueberry topping or fresh fruit.

Breakfast Tips

Ready, set, oats! Get oats into your morning in any form you like. Oats are found in the majority of our breakfasts, so if you are rotating through different breakfast recipes, make sure you're eating oats the majority of the time. Be bold and brave—try different preparations: savory oats, sweet oats, raw oats, cooked oats, and steel-cut oats. Try them in pancakes, try them in waffles, try them with fruit, or try them just plain. Oats are a winning way to start your day!

Make yourself a heaping helping of breakfast each morning. Many people find that preparing their oatmeal the night before works well. It can be heated up in the microwave or on the stovetop, and leftovers will keep well for several days! See the "Batch Cooking" section (pages 185–193) for ideas about the most efficient way to get a hearty breakfast every morning.

Think greens! Think about adding spinach or other greens to your morning meal. This may be a new concept for you, but you'll be adding meganutrients to your morning! Some of you may even become bold lovers of morning kale. Check out the Dressings and Topping Tips (page 267) to wake up your morning greens with flavor.

You won't find any smoothie or juice recipes here. Instead, you'll eat and enjoy whole fruits in their intact form. Slicing and peeling whole fruit is totally fine—just don't blend it or puree it in the food processor so that you can swallow it in one gulp. Indulge in a few pieces of glorious, ripe, whole fruit and your taste buds, stomach, and blood sugar levels will thank you.

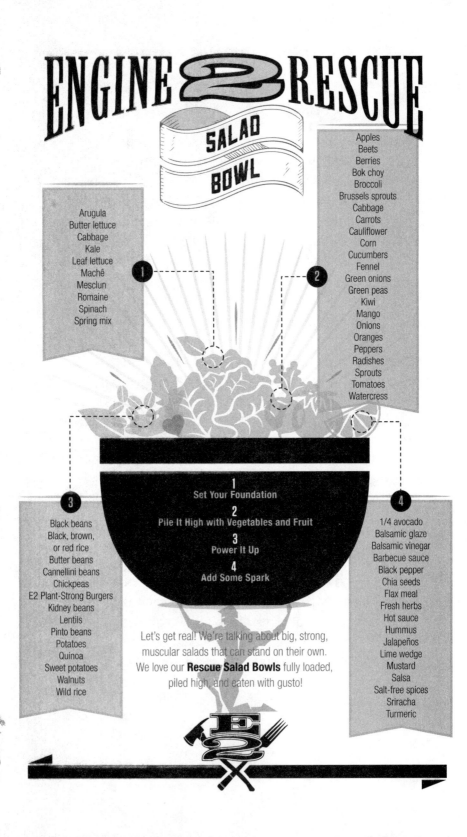

ENGINE 2 RESCUE
SALAD BOWL

Apples
Beets
Berries
Bok choy
Broccoli
Brussels sprouts
Cabbage
Carrots
Cauliflower
Corn
Cucumbers
Fennel
Green onions
Green peas
Kiwi
Mango
Onions
Oranges
Peppers
Radishes
Sprouts
Tomatoes
Watercress

Arugula
Butter lettuce
Cabbage
Kale
Leaf lettuce
Machê
Mesclun
Romaine
Spinach
Spring mix

1

2

1
Set Your Foundation

2
Pile It High with Vegetables and Fruit

3
Power It Up

4
Add Some Spark

3

Black beans
Black, brown,
or red rice
Butter beans
Cannellini beans
Chickpeas
E2 Plant-Strong Burgers
Kidney beans
Lentils
Pinto beans
Potatoes
Quinoa
Sweet potatoes
Walnuts
Wild rice

4

1/4 avocado
Balsamic glaze
Balsamic vinegar
Barbecue sauce
Black pepper
Chia seeds
Flax meal
Fresh herbs
Hot sauce
Hummus
Jalapeños
Lime wedge
Mustard
Salsa
Salt-free spices
Sriracha
Turmeric

Let's get real! We're talking about big, strong,
muscular salads that can stand on their own.
We love our **Rescue Salad Bowls** fully loaded,
piled high, and eaten with gusto!

LUNCH

Rescue Salad Bowls

Let's get real! We aren't talking about rabbit food here—like those tiny, silly salads made of lettuce, carrot shreds, and a tomato wedge. No sirree bob! We're talking about big, strong salads that can stand on their own for any meal: breakfast, lunch, or dinner. We love our salad bowls fully loaded, piled high and eaten with gusto!

Building Your Rescue Salad Bowls

SET YOUR FOUNDATION . . .

Arugula

Butter lettuce

Cabbage (red or green)

Kale

Leaf lettuce

Machê

Mesclun

Romaine

Spinach

Spring mix

THEN PILE IT HIGH WITH VEGETABLES AND FRUIT . . .

Apples

Beets

Berries

Bok choy

Broccoli

Brussels sprouts

Cabbage, red or green

Carrots

Cauliflower

Corn

Cucumbers

Fennel

Green onions

Green peas
Kiwi
Mango
Onions
Oranges
Peppers (bell or hot)
Radishes
Tomatoes
Sprouts (broccoli, radish, alfalfa)
Watercress

POWER IT UP WITH . . .

Black beans
Butter beans
Cannellini beans
Chickpeas
Engine 2 Plant-Strong Plant Burgers
Kidney beans
Lentils
Pinto beans
Potatoes
Quinoa
Rice (black, brown, or red, or a combination)
Sweet potatoes
Walnuts
Wild rice

ADD SOME SPARK . . .

Avocado (¼ avocado maximum per serving)
Balsamic glaze
Balsamic vinegar
Barbecue sauce
Black pepper
Chia seeds
Flax meal
Fresh herbs
Hot sauce

Hummus
Jalapeños
Lime wedge
Mustard
Salsa
Salt-free spices
Sriracha or other hot sauce
Turmeric

Check out the "Dressings, Hummus, Toppings, and Sides" section (see page 257) for seven amazing salad dressing ideas.

Rip's Favorite Salad: In a big bowl, lay a foundation of finely chopped dinosaur (lacinato) kale and romaine lettuce; then pile high with shredded beets, chopped apples, frozen roasted corn (thawed), diced red bell pepper, chopped and toasted walnuts, crumbled-up Engine 2 Pinto Habanero Plant Burger; and top with a spark of ¼ of an avocado, sliced, and the Sweet Fire Dressing on page 258.

Here are seven killer salad bowl recipes we can't gorge on enough!

Chopped and Cubed Salad

This salad is filling and fast to throw together, especially if your sweet potato is cooked ahead of time.

Serves 2

INGREDIENTS:

1 head romaine lettuce, chopped
1 sweet potato, cooked and cubed
½ mango, cubed
½ cup cooked kidney beans, drained and rinsed if canned

½ cup corn (fresh or thawed from frozen)
Fresh basil or cilantro, chopped
½ cup Sesame Seed Dressing (page 257) or dressing of choice

INSTRUCTIONS:

In a salad bowl, combine the romaine, sweet potato, mango, kidney beans, corn, and basil. Dress, toss, and serve.

All-Day Kale Salad

Once you trip the greens-for-breakfast wire, it changes your wiring for good! Jane often has veggies for breakfast, and Rip sometimes bypasses the big bowl of oats for a hearty morning salad. It's a compelling start to the day and gives you all the breakfast greens you'll ever need. Give it a try anytime of the day!

Serves 2 to 4

INGREDIENTS:

4 cups kale (about one bunch), leaves stripped from the spines and finely chopped

½ avocado, peeled and pitted (allow ¼ avocado maximum per serving)

4 ounces hummus, Engine 2–approved with no added tahini or oil

Juice of 1 lemon

2 green onions, diced

8 to 12 ounces canned mandarin oranges (ideally in their own juice, not syrup), drained and rinsed

INSTRUCTIONS:

Place the kale leaves in a large bowl, then add the avocado, hummus, and the lemon juice. Really massage the ingredients together (by squeezing hard) until the kale is dark green and reduced in size by half. Top with green onions and mandarin oranges and enjoy.

Gallo Pinto Salad

We adore Gallo Pinto! It's a traditional Costa Rican dish: black beans and rice. We then mix it together with a little salsa to amp up the plant power. Gracias, Costa Rica!

Note: Prep time can be a snap if using leftover rice, beans, and veggies from a Brown Rice Bowl meal (page 235).

Serves 2 to 4

INGREDIENTS:

1 to 2 cups cooked brown rice
1 to 2 cups cooked black beans,
    drained and rinsed if canned
½ cup shredded lettuce
½ cup cherry tomatoes, halved
½ cup shredded carrots
½ cup frozen sweet corn

¼ cup chopped green onion
½ cup diced red bell pepper
½ cup chopped cilantro (optional)
½ to 1 avocado, diced (allow ¼
    avocado maximum per serving)
Salsa
Balsamic vinegar

INSTRUCTIONS:

To a medium-size bowl, add the brown rice, black beans, lettuce, toma-toes, carrots, corn, green onion, pepper, cilantro (if using), avocado, and as much of your favorite salsa as you desire. Gently stir everything together until well mixed. Drizzle with balsamic vinegar to taste. Serve alongside a huge green salad or a pile of cooked greens.

Cro-Magnon Man Salad

Jane's husband loves to harvest this salad from the family's garden and yard like a true Cro-Magnon man. Yes! Jane and Brian have apple trees in their backyard! (Note: These ingredients are also available at your local grocery store.)

Serves 2

INGREDIENTS:

6 to 8 ounces mixed salad greens
1 small apple, diced
½ cup cooked wild rice
2 tablespoons dried cranberries

¼ cup raw pumpkin seeds,
    toasted
½ cup Sweet Fire Dressing (page
    258) or dressing of choice

INSTRUCTIONS:

In your most caveman-like wooden bowl, combine the mixed greens, apple, rice, cranberries, and pumpkin seeds. Dress, toss, and devour, utensils optional!

Yes Yes Yes Salad

Napa cabbage, kale, toasted walnuts and a sweet, fiery dressing combine to make this spectacular salad, and "Yes" is all we have to say. Yes. Yes. Yes.

Serves 2 to 4

INGREDIENTS:

2 cups kale, leaves stripped from the spines and chopped into thin, fine strips

½ Napa cabbage, chopped into thin, fine strips

¼ cup walnuts

1 (8-ounce) can mandarin oranges (ideally in their own juice, not syrup), drained and rinsed

1 avocado, mashed or cubed (allow ¼ avocado maximum per serving)

1 teaspoon lemon juice

½ to ¾ cup Sweet Fire Dressing (page 258) or other dressing of choice

INSTRUCTIONS:

Place the kale and Napa cabbage strips in a large bowl.

In a toaster oven or regular oven, toast the walnuts at 350°F for 4 to 5 minutes, or until fragrant and slightly browned. Watch closely! Set aside to cool.

Add the mandarin oranges, avocado, and lemon juice to the kale and Napa cabbage. Pour on the dressing and toss until all the ingredients are well coated. Serve yourself a heaping helping—or eat it right out of the big bowl!

Bellissima Pasta Salad

One of our first Seven-Day Rescue rock star participants, Char Nolan, is always presenting us with wonderful flavors from Italy. She grew up with these lovely ingredients from the Old Country: arugula, broccolini, cannellini, oregano, rosemary, basil, and on and on. Here is her Bellissima Pasta Salad.

Serves 2 to 4

INGREDIENTS:

6 ounces baby arugula, spinach, or spring mix

1 cup Roasted Red Peppers (page 266)

1 head broccolini, finely chopped

½ cup cooked cannellini beans, drained and rinsed if canned

1 cup cooked whole wheat rotini pasta

1 tomato, diced

¼ white onion, diced

1 clove garlic, minced

½ teaspoon dried rosemary

½ teaspoon dried oregano

½ teaspoon dried basil, or 1 teaspoon fresh basil

2 tablespoons red wine vinegar

2 shakes crushed red pepper flakes

INSTRUCTIONS:

In a large bowl, combine all the ingredients and toss. Serve to cheers of "Deliziosa!"

The Great Summer Novel Salad

This wild rice, arugula, and apricot salad is like a great summer novel: light, lingering, and sad when it is finished. You're left wanting more.

Serves 4

INGREDIENTS:

1 cup wild rice, cooked as directed (yields 3 cups cooked wild rice)
1½ cups red grapes, halved
3 green onions, chopped
½ cup finely sliced carrots
4 dried apricots, finely minced
1 red ancient sweet pepper (or red bell pepper), diced

½ cup toasted walnuts
6 to 8 fresh basil leaves, finely minced
1 cup Walnut Garlic Dressing (page 259)
2 cups arugula, torn into 2-inch pieces

INSTRUCTIONS:

Cook the wild rice per package instructions. Set aside and let cool.

In a large bowl, combine the wild rice, grapes, green onion, carrots, apricots, pepper, walnuts, and basil. Add the dressing and toss well.

Serve on big beds of arugula.

ENGINE 2 RESCUE

FLATS

★ ★ ★

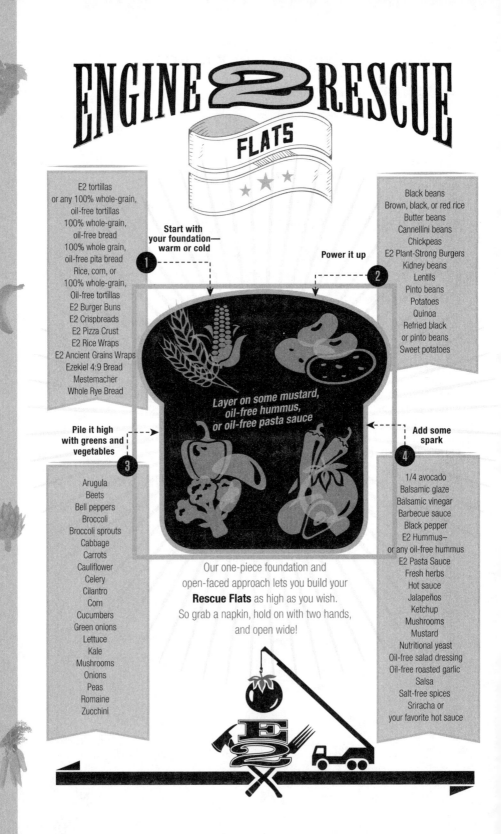

Start with your foundation— warm or cold ①

E2 tortillas
or any 100% whole-grain, oil-free tortillas
100% whole-grain, oil-free bread
100% whole grain, oil-free pita bread
Rice, corn, or 100% whole-grain, oil-free tortillas
E2 Burger Buns
E2 Crispbreads
E2 Pizza Crust
E2 Rice Wraps
E2 Ancient Grains Wraps
Ezekiel 4:9 Bread
Mestemacher Whole Rye Bread

Power it up ②

Black beans
Brown, black, or red rice
Butter beans
Cannellini beans
Chickpeas
E2 Plant-Strong Burgers
Kidney beans
Lentils
Pinto beans
Potatoes
Quinoa
Refried black or pinto beans
Sweet potatoes

Layer on some mustard, oil-free hummus, or oil-free pasta sauce

Pile it high with greens and vegetables ③

Arugula
Beets
Bell peppers
Broccoli
Broccoli sprouts
Cabbage
Carrots
Cauliflower
Celery
Cilantro
Corn
Cucumbers
Green onions
Lettuce
Kale
Mushrooms
Onions
Peas
Romaine
Zucchini

Add some spark ④

1/4 avocado
Balsamic glaze
Balsamic vinegar
Barbecue sauce
Black pepper
E2 Hummus— or any oil-free hummus
E2 Pasta Sauce
Fresh herbs
Hot sauce
Jalapeños
Ketchup
Mushrooms
Mustard
Nutritional yeast
Oil-free salad dressing
Oil-free roasted garlic
Salsa
Salt-free spices
Sriracha or your favorite hot sauce

Our one-piece foundation and open-faced approach lets you build your **Rescue Flats** as high as you wish. So grab a napkin, hold on with two hands, and open wide!

Rescue Flats

So many of us grew up on sandwiches that we understand why many people say, "Hey, I want something with bread!" So here's the answer: Flats! Our one-piece-of-bread, open-faced approach lets you build yours as high as you wish. If you drool at the thought of a big, juicy sandwich for lunch, or seek a dynamite dinner after a long day at work, here's to you, your flats, and your two hands you'll be using to eat them!

Building Your Rescue Flats

START WITH YOUR FOUNDATION—WARM OR COLD...

Engine 2 Tortillas—or any 100 percent whole-grain, oil-free tortillas

100 percent whole-grain, oil-free bread

100 percent whole-grain, oil-free pita bread

Rice, corn, or 100 percent whole-grain, oil-free tortillas

Engine 2 Burger Buns

Engine 2 Crispbreads

Engine 2 Pizza Crust

Engine 2 Rice Wraps

Engine 2 Ancient Grains Wraps

Ezekiel 4:9 Bread

Mestemacher Whole Rye Bread

LAYER ON SOME...

Mustard

Oil-free hummus

Oil-free pasta sauce

POWER IT UP WITH...

Black beans

Butter beans

Cannellini beans

Chickpeas

Engine 2 Plant-Strong Burgers

Kidney beans

Lentils

Pinto beans
Potatoes
Quinoa
Refried black or pinto beans
Rice (black, brown, or red, or a combination)
Sweet potatoes

PILE IT HIGH WITH GREENS AND VEGETABLES ...

Arugula
Beets
Bell peppers
Broccoli
Broccoli sprouts
Cabbage (red or green)
Carrots
Cauliflower
Celery
Cilantro
Corn
Cucumbers
Green onions
Lettuce
Kale
Mushrooms
Onions
Peas
Romaine
Zucchini

ADD SOME SPARK ...

Avocado (¼ avocado maximum per serving)
Balsamic glaze
Balsamic vinegar
Barbecue sauce
Black pepper
Fresh herbs
Hot sauce
Hummus (Engine 2 or any oil-free brand)

Jalapeños
    Ketchup
    Mushrooms
    Mustard
    Nutritional yeast
    Oil-free salad dressing
    Oil-free roasted garlic
    Pasta sauce (Engine 2 or any oil-free brand)
    Salsa
    Salt-free spices
    Sriracha or another hot sauce of your choice

Build your flat as high as you wish; let it overflow onto your plate. Serve it open-faced and cold if it's bread. Wrap it or fold it if it's a tortilla—then heat it, bake it, and eat it with your hands, with a fork, or over the sink!

Rip's Favorite Rescue Flat: Foundation of an Engine 2 Brown Rice Tortilla (first heated up in a skillet, 15 seconds on each side), layered with several gobs of hummus and refried black beans, topped with chopped curly kale, arugula, and cucumbers, with a spark of ¼ avocado and sriracha sauce! I always make two of these bountiful burritos.

Here are seven flat recipes we love opening our mouths wide and chomping into!

Good Breads, Buns, and Tortillas for Flats

When shopping for breads, we always look for any of the Ezekiel 4:9 or sprouted breads, 100 percent whole wheat bread, or 100 percent rye bread (we prefer Mestemacher brand).

For gluten-free options, try Engine 2 Brown Rice Tortillas or purchase Millet and Flax Bread from Sami's Bakery at samisbakery.com.

Food for Life and Engine 2 make whole-grain burger buns and whole-grain tortillas as well.

For pizza crust, Engine 2 has a 100 percent whole wheat version; for a gluten-free option, try the Millet and Flax Pizza Crust from Sami's Bakery at samisbakery.com.

Hummus and Avocado Flat

This is our classic flat, our go-to lunch or evening snack. These ingredients are easily found in the store, quick to layer on a flat, and fast at making your friends jealous. Keep your eye on your flat!

Makes 2 open-faced sandwiches

INGREDIENTS:

8 ounces Our Hummus (page 260) or any Engine 2 Seven-Day Rescue approved hummus with no tahini or added oil

2 or more slices 100 percent whole-grain bread

½ avocado, thinly sliced or mashed (allow ¼ avocado maximum per sandwich)

1 cucumber, sliced

1 tomato, sliced

Drizzle of balsamic glaze (we prefer Isola brand, Classic Cream of Balsamic—deceptively named as there is no cream in this product!)

4 romaine lettuce leaves, chopped or whole

INSTRUCTIONS:

Spread the hummus as thick as you wish on whichever bread you are using. Add the avocado and as many slices of cucumber and tomato as will fit on your sandwich. Drizzle an artistic zigzag of balsamic glaze over it all, top with romaine leaves for a good handhold, and enjoy.

Dip any leftover veggies into any leftover hummus if you find yourself needing a bit more at the end of lunch.

Black Bean and Sprouts Flat

The power of these wee little sprouts is breathtaking. We all know broccoli is good for us, but 1 ounce of broccoli sprouts has 10 to 100 times the cancer-protective compounds—sulforaphanes—as 1½ pounds of broccoli. How about that—just topping off your sandwich with an ounce of sulforaphane-containing broccoli sprouts will help your liver detoxify carcinogens!

Makes 2 open-faced sandwiches

INGREDIENTS:

½ cup cooked black beans, drained and rinsed if canned
2 to 4 tablespoons brown mustard
2 or more slices 100 percent whole-grain bread
1 cucumber, sliced

1 tomato, sliced
Handful of broccoli sprouts
Drizzle of balsamic glaze or a bit of mustard
4 romaine lettuce leaves, chopped or whole, if using

INSTRUCTIONS:

Pour the black beans into a bowl. Using the backside of a fork, mash at least half of the beans until their skins break. (When they are semi-mashed, they stay on the sandwich better.) Set aside.

Spread your favorite brown mustard as thick as you wish on whichever bread you are using. On top add the cucumber, tomato, sprouts, and black beans. Drizzle balsamic glaze on top for a sweet kick. If necessary, top with romaine leaves for a good handhold, and enjoy.

Dip any leftover veggies into any leftover mustard if you find yourself needing a bit more at the end of lunch.

Black Bean Hummus and Tomatoes Flat

Black beans are champions! Not only of flavor, but of fiber, folate, protein, and iron. Make hummus with black beans a Seven-Day Rescue champion for all those reasons and more!

Makes 2 open-faced sandwiches

INGREDIENTS:

8 ounces Black Bean Hummus (page 261) or any Engine 2 Seven-Day Rescue approved hummus with no tahini or added oil

2 or more slices 100 percent whole-grain bread or other recommended bread (see Good Breads, Buns, and Tortillas for Flats on page 219)

1 cup fresh spinach

1 cucumber, sliced

1 cup cherry tomatoes, sliced in half (or 1 tomato, sliced)

Drizzle of balsamic glaze or a bit of mustard

4 romaine lettuce leaves, chopped or whole, if using

INSTRUCTIONS:

Spread the black bean hummus as thick as you wish on whichever bread you're using. Add a layer of spinach, cucumber slices, and as many cherry tomatoes as will fit on your sandwich. Drizzle balsamic glaze over it all, top with romaine leaves if necessary for a good handhold, and enjoy. This sandwich can be a bear of a mess, and the lettuce on top will serve as the top of the sandwich to help you get a better hold on it.

Dip any leftover veggies into any leftover hummus if you find yourself needing a bit more at the end of lunch.

Red Pepper Smile Flat

This bountiful sandwich made with both red pepper hummus and roasted red peppers is bound to make your stomach happy, make your friends want bites, and make everyone smile! (For a nutritional analysis of a Red Pepper Smile Flat vs. a bologna-and-cheese sandwich, see page 287.)

Makes 2 open-faced sandwiches

INGREDIENTS:

8 ounces Red Pepper Hummus (page 261) or any Engine 2 Seven-Day Rescue approved hummus with no tahini or added oil

2 or more slices 100 percent whole-grain bread or other recommended bread (see Good Breads, Buns, and Tortillas for Flats on page 219)

¼ cup parsley, loosely chopped

4 green onions, chopped

½ cup Roasted Red Peppers (page 266) or store-bought (look for low-sodium and no added oil)

1 to 2 handfuls of fresh spinach leaves

1 tomato, sliced

Drizzle of balsamic glaze or a bit of mustard

4 romaine lettuce leaves, chopped or whole, if using

INSTRUCTIONS:

Spread the red pepper hummus as thick as you wish on whichever bread you've chosen. Add the parsley, green onion, roasted red peppers, spinach, and tomato. Drizzle balsamic glaze over it all. If necessary, top with romaine leaves for a good handhold, and enjoy.

Dip any leftover veggies into any leftover hummus if you find yourself needing a bit more at the end of lunch.

Sweet Potato Hummus and Chickpeas Flat

The sweet potato hummus used in this recipe is offered at the Cleveland Clinic Prevent and Reverse Heart Disease Seminar conducted by our parents. People swoon over this hummus, which seems to serve as some sort of healing balm. Anything tastes good on the foundation of sweet potato hummus—here is our favorite recipe that uses it, but you can get creative and experiment with other combinations if you'd like.

Makes 2 open-faced sandwiches

INGREDIENTS:

½ cup cooked chickpeas, drained and rinsed if canned

8 ounces Sweet Potato Convert Hummus (page 262) or any Engine 2 Seven-Day Rescue approved hummus with no tahini or added oil

2 or more slices 100 percent whole-grain bread or other recommended bread (see Good Breads, Buns, and Tortillas for Flats on page 219)

4 green onions, chopped

1 to 2 handfuls of fresh spinach leaves

1 tomato, sliced

½ avocado, thinly sliced or mashed (allow ¼ avocado maximum per sandwich)

¼ cup loosely packed cilantro (or parsley, whatever kind you like)

Drizzle of balsamic glaze or a bit of mustard

4 romaine lettuce leaves, chopped or whole, if using

INSTRUCTIONS:

Pour the chickpeas into a bowl. Using the backside of a fork, mash at least half of the peas until their skins break. (When they are semi-mashed, they'll stay on the sandwich better.) Set aside.

Spread the sweet potato hummus as thick as you wish on whichever bread you use. Add the green onion, chickpeas, spinach, tomato, avocado, and cilantro. Drizzle balsamic glaze over it all, top with romaine leaves if necessary for a good handhold, and enjoy.

Dip any leftover veggies into any leftover hummus if you find yourself needing a bit more at the end of lunch.

Red Pepper and Arugula Flat

Arugula is a spicy, feisty green that bites back! Once you fall in love with it, you will be hooked.

Makes 2 open-faced sandwiches

INGREDIENTS:

8 ounces Red Pepper Hummus (page 261) or any Engine 2 Seven-Day Rescue approved hummus with no tahini or added oil
2 or more slices 100 percent whole-grain bread or other recommended bread (see Good Breads, Buns, and Tortillas for Flats on page 219)
1 to 2 handfuls of fresh arugula
1 tomato, sliced

½ avocado, thinly sliced or mashed (allow ¼ avocado maximum per sandwich)
½ cup Roasted Red Pepper strips (page 266) or store-bought (look for low-sodium and no added oil)
Drizzle of balsamic glaze or a bit of mustard
4 romaine lettuce leaves, chopped or whole, if using

INSTRUCTIONS:

Spread the red pepper hummus as thick as you wish on whichever bread you choose. Add the arugula, tomato, avocado, and roasted red peppers. Drizzle balsamic glaze over it all, top with romaine leaves if necessary for a good handhold, and enjoy.

Dip any leftover veggies into any leftover hummus if you find yourself needing a bit more at the end of lunch.

Salad-Topped Pizza Flat

Two all-time favorites here: fresh salad and warm pizza! Once this pizza comes out of the oven, throw the salad on top, slice, and enjoy! Engine 2 Pizza Crusts are available at Whole Foods Market stores across the country. They are made with 100 percent whole wheat, naturally sweetened with a touch of maple syrup, and stone-oven baked for an authentic pizzeria taste. They are the perfect foundation for a plant-strong pizza! They can be found in either the freezer section or the pasta sauce section. Ask a Whole Foods Market team member for help and tell them Rip sent you!

For a gluten-free option, order your crust ahead of time at samisbakery.com.

Note—please read the recipe directions carefully—the salad goes on top after the pizza crust is cooked.

Makes one 12-inch pizza

INGREDIENTS:

1 whole-grain pizza crust (such as Engine 2 Pizza Crust or another brand that works for Engine 2 guidelines—or see the box below to make your own)

1½ to 2 cups no-oil-added pasta sauce

3 medium tomatoes, thinly sliced

3 tablespoons nutritional yeast

2 cups fresh spinach, chopped

2 cups arugula or romaine, chopped

2 green onions, chopped

½ cup pineapple, cubed, fresh, or canned in its own juice and drained (optional)

1 red pepper, chopped

1 to 2 tablespoons lemon juice

INSTRUCTIONS:

Prepare the Pizza Crust:

Preheat the oven to 400°F. Line a baking sheet with parchment paper.

Place the pizza crust on the lined pan. Bake for 4 to 5 minutes, or until the crust gets warm, slightly browned, and crisp (or according to package directions).

Prepare the Pizza:

Onto the warm crust, pour the pasta sauce and spread evenly. Arrange the tomato slices on the sauce. Sprinkle the tomatoes with nutritional yeast and place the crust back in the oven for 15 to 20 minutes.

Prepare the Salad:

In a bowl, combine the spinach, arugula (or romaine), green onion, pineapple (if using), and red pepper. Sprinkle lemon juice over the salad and toss well. Set aside—this is NOT to be cooked on the pizza.

Build Your Salad Pizza:

Remove the pizza from the oven and transfer the fresh salad right on top of it in a big heap!

Slice up this beauty and serve along with a green salad or a heaping helping of cooked greens.

Tip: Many people love fresh salad on top of cooked pizza. But if you have other ideas for healthy pizza toppings, indulge your imagination and your taste buds!

Make Your Own Pizza Crust!

If you want to make your own crust, here is J. R.'s Pizza Crust recipe from *Plant-Strong*:

  3 cups whole wheat flour, plus 1 cup for coating work
    surface and baking pans
  1 packet active dry yeast
  ⅛ teaspoon salt (optional)
  ½ cup unsweetened applesauce
  1¼ cups warm water

Instructions:
In a large bowl, blend together the flour, yeast, and salt, if using. Add the applesauce and water and stir in with

a large spoon or fork until the mixture forms a ball of dough. Knead the dough ball on a flat working surface or right in the bowl until the dough tension increases. Add additional flour to your work surface and the outside of the dough as needed if it is sticky.

Cover the dough ball with a damp paper towel and set aside to rise for 10 minutes.

Preheat the oven to 400°F.

Divide the dough into 4 to 6 equal-size hunks, depending on the desired size of pizza crust. Knead each piece of dough into a firm ball; cover with a clean, damp cloth; and let rise for 10 minutes. Flatten out the dough by hand or with a rolling pin to the desired crust thickness; then, using a fork, poke numerous holes in it to limit crust bubbles. Bake on a flour-coated baking sheet, parchment paper–lined pan, or pizza stone.

The crusts can be baked with or without toppings—the time will vary depending on the thickness of the dough. Bake time is usually 5 minutes for a thin crust without toppings; 15 to 20 minutes for a thicker crust with toppings.

Rescue Soup Bowls

Split Pea Potato Soup

This soup brings back old memories of days gone by. Jane used to write her college essays weekend after weekend while eating this comforting bowl. Serve this hearty soup alone, or over penne pasta, brown rice, or, if you prefer, quinoa. Go for it!

Serves 6

INGREDIENTS:

6 cups low-sodium vegetable broth or water
1½ cups dry split peas

1 bay leaf
½ teaspoon dry mustard
1 onion, chopped

2 cloves garlic, minced
2 celery stalks, chopped
2 carrots, chopped
3 medium red-skinned potatoes, cubed
1 tablespoon low-sodium tamari

1 tablespoon balsamic vinegar
Black pepper
Hot sauce
Parsley (whatever kind you like), chopped, for garnish

INSTRUCTIONS:

In a large soup pot over high heat, mix the broth (or water), split peas, bay leaf, and mustard. Bring to a boil, then lower heat to a simmer for about 20 minutes while partially covered.

Add the onion, garlic, celery, carrots, and potatoes. Cover and simmer for about 40 minutes more, stirring occasionally, until the peas are creamy.

Toward the end of the cooking time add the tamari, vinegar, and black pepper to taste. As the peas cook, their texture becomes creamier and softer and the stirring blends them.

Serve in big soup bowls garnished with your favorite hot sauce and parsley, along with a huge green salad or a pile of cooked greens.

Lemon Lentil Soup

Jane made this soup one afternoon for dinner, and before she knew it, Rip had devoured all four servings! It's that good. Make it your own by adjusting the amount of lemon, cilantro, and spices. In fact, we often double the recipe when we make it so that we can eat double amounts!

Serves 4

INGREDIENTS:

1 cup brown rice, uncooked (optional)
1 large onion, chopped
6 cloves garlic, chopped
2 tablespoons tomato paste
¼ teaspoon ground cumin
¼ teaspoon chili powder
Pinch of cayenne pepper
¼ teaspoon black pepper
6 cups vegetable broth

1½ cups red lentils
3 large carrots, diced
1 to 2 cups chopped stems and leaves of beet greens or Swiss chard
2 tablespoons lemon juice
Zest of 1 lemon
1 cup cilantro or parsley (whatever kind you like)

INSTRUCTIONS:

If using, prepare brown rice per the package instructions. Set aside. Or use 2 cups frozen brown rice, prepared as directed.

In a soup pot over medium heat, cook the onion until beginning to brown, about 5 minutes. Add splashes of water if necessary. Add the garlic and cook, stirring constantly, for 2 more minutes. Add the tomato paste, cumin, chili powder, cayenne, and black pepper and cook for another minute while the spices integrate. Add the vegetable broth, lentils, and carrots and bring to a boil. Turn the heat to simmer, partially cover, and cook about 10 minutes, or until the lentils and carrots are starting to soften. Add the beet stems and greens and cook for another 20 minutes.

We like the soup chunky, but if you wish, purée some with an immersion blender right in the pot or put some in a blender. Stir the lemon juice and lemon zest into the soup and garnish with cilantro. Serve with a scoop of brown rice, if using, alongside a huge green salad or a pile of cooked greens.

Southwest Stew

This rich, satisfying stew freezes well and is great to make ahead of time for family and friends. Don't be alarmed by what looks like a long list of ingredients—they are mostly spices!

Serves 4

INGREDIENTS:

1 onion, chopped
2 cloves garlic, minced
1 poblano pepper, diced
1 orange bell pepper, diced
2 cups cubed butternut squash (buy cubed squash, or bake a whole squash at 350°F for 1 hour, then peel and cube)
1 tablespoon ground cumin
1 teaspoon chili powder
1 teaspoon garlic powder
1 teaspoon onion powder
¼ teaspoon cayenne pepper
1 (15-ounce) can fire-roasted tomatoes

3 cups low-sodium vegetable broth
1 dry chipotle pepper, soaked in water overnight (or until soft), drained and minced
1 (15-ounce) can black beans, drained and rinsed
1 cup frozen white sweet corn
1 cup cooked brown rice (frozen works well here)
5 ounces baby spinach leaves
Juice of 1 lime
½ bunch cilantro, leaves and tender stems chopped
¼ teaspoon salt (optional)

INSTRUCTIONS:

Warm a medium soup pot over medium-high heat until water sprinkled on the surface bubbles and jumps. Add the onion, garlic, poblano pepper, orange bell pepper, and butternut squash and cook for 5 minutes while stirring. Add the cumin, chili powder, garlic powder, onion powder, and cayenne pepper and stir for about 1 minute more. Add the tomatoes, broth, chipotle, black beans, corn, and brown rice. Bring to a boil, then reduce the heat to a simmer for about 30 minutes, or until the butternut squash is tender. Add the spinach leaves, lime juice, cilantro, and the salt, if using. Cook 1 to 2 minutes more, or until the spinach wilts. Ladle the stew into bowls, add a scoop of brown rice, and enjoy along with a huge green salad, a pile of cooked greens, or broccoli, asparagus, or green beans—whatever you'd like.

Miso Barley Soup

This has been one of Jane's favorites since she met her husband, Brian, twenty-five years ago. It was one of the food potions he won her over with! This soup is great for lunch or dinner and, apparently, romance.

Serves 4

INGREDIENTS:

2½ cups water
¾ cup hulled barley
1 small onion, diced
2 celery stalks, chopped
4 ounces mushrooms, sliced
1 red bell pepper, diced
1 zucchini, diced

1 small sweet potato, peeled and diced
2½ cups low-sodium vegetable stock
2 tablespoons white miso
1 teaspoon garlic powder
2 tablespoons port or white wine (optional)

INSTRUCTIONS:

In a small pan over high heat, mix the water and barley. Bring to a boil, then reduce to a simmer for about 1 hour, or until all the liquid is absorbed.

In a soup pot over medium-high heat, cook the onion, celery, and mushrooms, stirring constantly, until the onion becomes translucent and the mushrooms appear thoroughly cooked. Add the pepper, zucchini, and sweet potato to the pot and continue stirring for 5 minutes.

Add the vegetable stock, barley, and miso. It is helpful to heat a cup of broth in the microwave, add in the miso, stir until dissolved, and then add the mixture to the pot. Stir in the garlic powder and port, if using, and continue cooking until the sweet potatoes are cooked through and the miso flavor has blended into all the ingredients, about 15 to 20 minutes.

Serve warm along with a huge green salad or a pile of cooked greens.

> I was never a big vegetable fan, but I was quite amazed how most of the food tasted. Before the Seven-Day Rescue, my wife could never get me to eat cucumbers, and she couldn't believe it when I did!
> —James McVeigh, age 68, retired city treasurer, North Ridgeville, Ohio

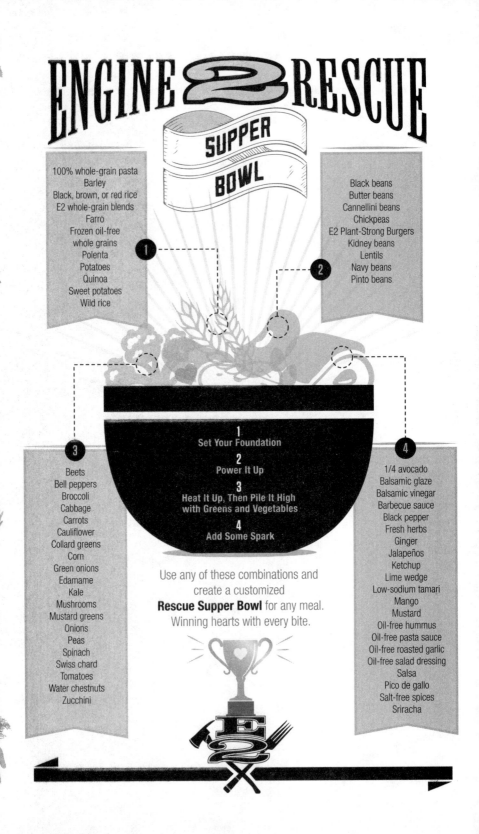

ENGINE 2 RESCUE

SUPPER BOWL

1
100% whole-grain pasta
Barley
Black, brown, or red rice
E2 whole-grain blends
Farro
Frozen oil-free
whole grains
Polenta
Potatoes
Quinoa
Sweet potatoes
Wild rice

2
Black beans
Butter beans
Cannellini beans
Chickpeas
E2 Plant-Strong Burgers
Kidney beans
Lentils
Navy beans
Pinto beans

3
Beets
Bell peppers
Broccoli
Cabbage
Carrots
Cauliflower
Collard greens
Corn
Green onions
Edamame
Kale
Mushrooms
Mustard greens
Onions
Peas
Spinach
Swiss chard
Tomatoes
Water chestnuts
Zucchini

1
Set Your Foundation

2
Power It Up

3
Heat It Up, Then Pile It High
with Greens and Vegetables

4
Add Some Spark

4
1/4 avocado
Balsamic glaze
Balsamic vinegar
Barbecue sauce
Black pepper
Fresh herbs
Ginger
Jalapeños
Ketchup
Lime wedge
Low-sodium tamari
Mango
Mustard
Oil-free hummus
Oil-free pasta sauce
Oil-free roasted garlic
Oil-free salad dressing
Salsa
Pico de gallo
Salt-free spices
Sriracha

Use any of these combinations and
create a customized
Rescue Supper Bowl for any meal.
Winning hearts with every bite.

DINNER

Rescue Supper Bowls

Bowls are in vogue for good reasons. They are visually appealing; you can layer, or place side by side, whatever ingredients you like; and all the flavors meld together, making every bite scintillating! Use any of these Rescue combinations and create a personal-size bowl for supper— and they also make a great lunch or breakfast. They are good to the last bite. Arguably, the saucy last bite is the best.

Building Your Rescue Supper Bowl

SET YOUR FOUNDATION . . .
    100 percent whole-grain pasta
    Barley
    Engine 2 whole-grain blends
    Farro
    Frozen oil-free whole grains
    Polenta
    Potatoes
    Quinoa
    Rice (black, brown, or red, or a combination)
    Sweet potatoes
    Wild rice

POWER IT UP WITH . . .
    Black beans
    Butter beans
    Cannellini beans
    Chickpeas
    Engine 2 Plant-Strong Burgers
    Kidney beans
    Lentils
    Navy beans
    Pinto beans

HEAT IT UP, THEN PILE IT HIGH WITH GREENS AND VEGETABLES ...

Beets

Bell peppers

Broccoli

Cabbage, red or green

Carrots

Cauliflower

Collard greens

Corn

Edamame

Green onions

Kale

Mushrooms

Mustard greens

Onions

Peas

Spinach

Swiss chard

Tomatoes

Water chestnuts

Zucchini

ADD SOME SPARK ...

Avocado (allow ¼ avocado maximum per serving)

Balsamic glaze

Balsamic vinegar

Barbecue sauce

Black pepper

Fresh herbs

Ginger

Jalapeños

Ketchup

Lime wedge

Low-sodium tamari

Mango

Mustard

Oil-free hummus
Oil-free pasta sauce
Oil-free roasted garlic
Oil-free salad dressing
Salsa
Pico de gallo
Salt-free spices
Sriracha

Rip's Favorite Supper Bowl: In a big bowl, lay a foundation of brown rice, power it up with black beans and pinto beans, pile high with diced tomatoes, green onions, bell peppers, corn, and water chestnuts, and then add a spark of pico de gallo, low-sodium tamari, and ¼ of an avocado.

Here are eight dinner bowl recipes we love to devour!

Brown Rice Bowl

This simple, tasty delight has been the mainstay of the Esselstyn family going back more than thirty years. No exaggeration, we have it at least twice a week, and it is an absolute must at all family gatherings of over twenty people. It's super economical, too. It was a firehouse favorite at Rip's old Station 2 because Rip could feed a crew of five hungry firefighters for under fifteen bucks! (For a nutritional analysis of a Brown Rice Bowl vs. a chicken Alfredo bowl, see page 287.)

Serves 2

INGREDIENTS:

1½ cups brown rice, uncooked
1 (15-ounce) can black beans, drained and rinsed
½ teaspoon ground cumin
½ teaspoon garlic powder
¼ teaspoon chili powder
1½ cups salsa, divided (½ cup for the beans and the rest for topping)

2 cups chopped romaine lettuce
(use prepared romaine from
a salad bag or chop 1 head of
romaine)
3 to 4 green onions, chopped

1 cup cherry tomatoes, halved
Hot sauce (we prefer sriracha)
¼ cup fresh cilantro, coarsely
chopped (optional)

INSTRUCTIONS:

Prepare the Rice:

If using frozen brown rice, prepare desired amount, around 2 to 4 cups, per package instructions, and skip to the next step of preparing the beans.

Or, in a rice cooker, prepare the rice per package instructions.

Or, in a pot over high heat, add 3 cups of water and 1½ cups of rice. When the rice and water come to a boil, turn the heat down to low, cover, and let simmer for about 40 minutes, or until all the water is absorbed and small steam holes are visible on the surface. When the rice is cooked and warm, it is time to make the beans.

Prepare the Beans:

Place the beans in a microwavable bowl and heat for 60 seconds. Or, if you prefer the stovetop, place the beans in a small pot over medium-high heat, stirring occasionally, for about 2 minutes, or until thoroughly warmed. Add the cumin, garlic powder, chili powder, and ½ cup of your favorite salsa to the beans and stir well. Set aside.

Build Your Brown Rice Bowl:

In the base of 2 large dinner bowls, place a layer of romaine lettuce followed by a layer each of brown rice, beans, green onion, and tomatoes; on top of it all add salsa, the hot sauce of your choice, and a garnish of cilantro, if using. Grab your fork, because you are ready to dive into your Brown Rice Bowl dinner! Don't forget to serve along with a green salad, other veggies, or a heaping helping of cooked greens.

Southwestern Potato Bowl

What is more filling than potatoes? And what packs more Southwestern flavor than Ro-Tel Diced Tomatoes and Green Chilies? Nothing and no one. So, giddyup! After gobbling up these taters topped with taste, you will feel like riding in a rodeo!

Serves 2

INGREDIENTS:

4 large Yukon Gold potatoes
1 (15-ounce) can pinto beans, drained, rinsed, and mashed
½ to 1 cup Ro-Tel Diced Tomatoes and Green Chilies (look for no- or low-salt versions)
8 ounces frozen corn (we prefer white corn as it is sweeter!)

1 red bell pepper, diced
2 green onions, chopped
2 to 4 cups fresh spinach
Fresh cilantro, for garnish
Hot sauce

INSTRUCTIONS:

Prepare the Yukon Gold Potatoes:

Prepare the Yukon Gold potatoes any way you prefer:

Microwave the potatoes, 2 at a time, for 8 to 10 minutes, or until each potato is soft and cooked through.

Or preheat the oven to 375°F. Place the potatoes directly on the oven rack. Bake for 45 minutes to 1 hour, or until soft and cooked through.

Prepare the Beans:

Place the beans in a microwavable bowl and heat for 60 seconds. Or, if you prefer the stovetop, place the beans in a small pot over medium-high heat, stirring occasionally, for about 2 minutes, or until thoroughly warmed. With the backside of a fork, smash about half of the beans. Add the desired amount of Ro-Tel tomatoes to the beans, along with the corn, pepper, and green onion. Set aside.

Build Your Southwestern Potato Bowl:

In the base of 2 large dinner bowls, place a layer of fresh spinach, followed by the potato, cut in half or cubed (your choice). Add the bean mixture on top of the potato and garnish with cilantro and a few shakes of your favorite hot sauce. Don't forget to serve along with a green salad or a heaping helping of cooked greens.

Sweet Potato Bowl

This is an absolute staple in Rip's life. In fact, he has a version of this bowl at least three times a week. He loves the nutrient-packed sweet potatoes dazzled with lime, mango, beans, and a little hot kick from the salsa. Sweet potatoes are one of the strongest foods around. They contain vitamin B_6, vitamin C, beta-carotene, vitamin D, potassium, iron, magnesium, calcium, protein, and fiber! Be sure to eat the skin as well. It is packed with power, fiber, and nutrients.

Serves 2

INGREDIENTS:

2 large sweet potatoes
1 (15-ounce) can black beans, drained and rinsed
¼ teaspoon ground cumin
¼ teaspoon garlic powder
¼ teaspoon chili powder
4 ounces mesclun mix (or fresh spinach)
4 to 6 green onions, chopped

1 mango, skinned and cubed (or 1 cup cubed frozen mango)
1 red pepper, chopped
½ avocado, mashed or diced (allow ¼ avocado maximum per serving)
¼ cup cilantro, chopped (optional)
Zest and juice of 1 lime
Salsa

INSTRUCTIONS:

Prepare the Sweet Potatoes:

Prepare the sweet potatoes any way you prefer: Microwave each whole sweet potato for about 8 minutes, or until soft. Or, preheat the oven to 400°F. Line a baking sheet with parchment paper. Bake the whole sweet potato on the lined pan in the oven for 45 minutes to 1 hour, or until soft.

Or, peel the sweet potato, cube it, and place in a steamer basket. Place at least 2 inches of water in the bottom of the steamer, cover, and steam the sweet potatoes for 8 to 10 minutes, or until thoroughly soft.

Prepare the Beans:

Place the beans in a microwavable bowl and heat for 60 seconds. Or, if you prefer the stovetop, place the beans in a small pot over medium-high heat, stirring occasionally, for about 2 minutes, or until warmed through. Add the cumin, garlic powder, and chili powder to the beans and stir well. Set aside.

Build Your Sweet Potato Bowl:

In the base of 2 large dinner bowls, place a layer of mesclun mix followed by the sweet potato—cut in half or cubed, your choice. On top of the sweet potato add the beans, green onion, mango, red pepper, avocado, cilantro, if using, and lime zest and juice. Add as much salsa of your choice as you wish. Don't forget to serve along with a green salad or a heaping helping of cooked greens.

Red Quinoa Bowl

Hats off to quinoa. Quinoa is a nutrient powerhouse of a grain. Actually, truth be told, it is technically a seed—a seed loaded with protein, iron, folate, fiber, and healthy omega-3 fatty acids! No wonder this ancient grain/seed from the Andes has made its way into our bowls. Be sure to cook your quinoa per package directions. Some brands need to be rinsed first to avoid a bitter taste. When cooked, quinoa should be soft but chewy, and the little roundish germ should be visible on top of the grains.

Serves 2

INGREDIENTS:

2 cups red quinoa, uncooked
1 (15-ounce) can cannellini beans, drained and rinsed
¼ red onion, diced
¼ teaspoon ground cumin
1 teaspoon lime juice (optional: add some lime zest)

2 cups butter lettuce leaves
½ cup pineapple chunks, fresh or canned in their own juice
1 red bell pepper, diced
½ cup Jane's Dancing Dressing (page 258)

INSTRUCTIONS:

Prepare the Quinoa:

In a rice cooker, prepare the quinoa as directed (some quinoa needs to be rinsed ahead of time to remove a bitter, soapy flavor, and some quinoa has already been prerinsed). Or, in a pot over high heat, add 4 cups of water and 2 cups of quinoa. When the quinoa and water come to a boil, turn the heat down to low, cover, and let simmer for 20 minutes. When the quinoa is cooked and warm, it is time to make the beans.

Prepare the Beans:

Place the beans in a microwavable bowl and heat for 60 seconds. Or, if you prefer the stovetop, place the beans in a small pot over medium-high heat, stirring occasionally, for about 2 minutes, or until warmed through. Add the onion, cumin, and lime juice and stir. Set aside.

Build Your Red Quinoa Bowl:

In the base of 2 large dinner bowls, place a layer of butter lettuce, followed by the quinoa and a layer each of beans, pineapple (and some of the juice, if you prefer), and red pepper. Top it all off with dressing. Grab your fork and dive into your Red Quinoa Bowl! Don't forget to serve along with a green salad or a heaping helping of cooked greens.

Mighty Green Pasta Bowl

Pasta is a quick and easy comfort food! Best of all, lots of companies now make 100 percent whole wheat pasta. Years ago, we had to drive across town to find a health food store that sold whole wheat pasta, whole wheat flour, and brown rice. That's hardly the case now! Also, there are fantastic gluten-free noodle options for those with sensitivities. And for those of you who own a spiralizer, making zucchini noodles is a wild and fun option.

Serves 2

INGREDIENTS:

12 ounces 100 percent whole wheat pasta, gluten-free pasta, or spiralized zucchini

3 cups kale, leaves stripped from spines and chopped into bite-size pieces

4 cups fresh spinach leaves

24 ounces pasta sauce (no added oil)

2 to 3 teaspoons nutritional yeast

¼ cup parsley, stems removed and coarsely chopped

INSTRUCTIONS:

Prepare the Pasta:

In a large pot over high heat, bring roughly 10 cups of water to a boil. Add the pasta for the number of minutes directed on the package. Set a timer for 3 minutes less than the package directions recommend. When the timer goes off, add the chopped kale to the pasta and water so it will cook along with the pasta for the last 3 minutes.

While the pasta and kale are cooking, pour the pasta sauce into a pan over medium heat and keep warm until ready to use.

When the timer goes off, drain the pasta and greens in a colander and set aside.

Build Your Pasta Bowl:

In the base of 2 large dinner bowls, place a layer of spinach, followed by a heaping pile of pasta and as much pasta sauce as you wish. Sprinkle nutritional yeast (this is similar to Parmesan cheese) over all and garnish with parsley. Enjoy with a huge green salad or a heaping helping of broccoli.

Empower Bowl

Wow! Even the name should get you fired up! Jane feels powerful just thinking about this lunch, and even more so after eating it. We both like to make the sweet potatoes and quinoa ahead of time so the salad is easy to put together at a moment's notice. This salad can be customized with any of your favorite fruits or vegetables.

Serves 2

INGREDIENTS:

1 large sweet potato, peeled and cubed
4 cups packed spinach
1 cup cooked quinoa
1 (15-ounce) can chickpeas, drained and rinsed
¼ cup toasted walnuts

1 apple, diced
½ cup red cabbage, finely chopped
½ avocado, diced
½ cup Sweet Fire Dressing (page 258)

INSTRUCTIONS:

Preheat the oven to 400°F. Line a large baking sheet with parchment paper.

Place the cubed sweet potatoes on the baking sheet and roast until tender, about 30 minutes.

In a large bowl, combine the spinach, roasted sweet potatoes, quinoa, chickpeas, toasted walnuts, apple, red cabbage, and avocado.

Drizzle the dressing over the salad and toss until everything is well coated. Serve up the power!

Mexican Polenta Bowl

Polenta is a nutrient-dense European dish made from finely ground cornmeal that is making its way onto our menus. The first time Rip had this dish was at the Muse School, a 100 percent plant-based, K–12 school in Malibu, California, founded by Suzy Cameron and her sister, Rebecca Amos. Students, teachers, and staff alike were all eating this goodness. Talk about smart moves.

Serves 4

INGREDIENTS:

1 cup dry polenta
¼ cup nutritional yeast
4 large cloves garlic, minced
½ teaspoon salt (optional)
2 jalapeño peppers, seeded and minced (divided)
4 cups water
1 (15-ounce) can black beans, drained and rinsed

2 tomatoes, diced
4 green onions, thinly sliced
½ cup cilantro, large stems removed
1 avocado, diced or mashed (allow ¼ avocado maximum per serving)
Juice of 1 to 2 limes

INSTRUCTIONS:

In a small bowl, combine the polenta, nutritional yeast, garlic, salt (if using), and 1 teaspoon jalapeño or more to taste.

In a medium pot, add the water and heat over medium-high heat until bubbles start to surface.

With a whisk in one hand and the bowl in the other, slowly pour the polenta mixture into the hot water—whisking all the while. Once all the polenta is added, the mixture will be thick and paste-like. Turn the heat to low. Whisk for about 5 minutes to ensure there are no lumps and the mixture is uniformly thickened.

Pour the polenta into 4 bowls and serve topped with black beans, tomatoes, green onion, cilantro, avocado, and a generous squeeze of fresh lime juice.

Thai Green Curry Bowl

We love Thai food! The blend of vegetables, spices, freshness, and the complement of flavors balanced with all the textures is dreamy...just like this Green Curry Bowl. We hope you love this as much as we do and that it becomes an easy (and healthy) way to satisfy your Thai food craving.

Serves 4 to 6

INGREDIENTS:

2 cups brown basmati rice, to yield 4 cups cooked
1 large onion, julienned
8 ounces mushrooms, sliced

2 heads of broccoli, cut into florets
1 red pepper, diced
2 carrots, sliced into thin rounds

1 (8-ounce) can baby corn, drained
   and rinsed (or use fresh)
2 cups unsweetened plain oat milk
1 teaspoon coconut extract
1 tablespoon maple syrup

2 to 3 teaspoons green curry
   paste (Thai Kitchen makes an
   oil-free brand)
6 to 8 leaves fresh basil, or Thai
   basil if available, finely chopped

INSTRUCTIONS:

Prepare the rice per package directions. Set aside.

In a large frying pan over high heat, cook the onion. Slowly reduce the heat as the onion browns, stirring continuously. Add the mushrooms, broccoli, red pepper, carrots, and baby corn; cover and cook until their colors turn bright and they still have snap. In a saucepan over medium-high heat, combine the oat milk, coconut extract, maple syrup, and curry paste. Stir until warm and well combined.

Pour over the cooked vegetables, and serve with the brown basmati rice and a garnish of basil. You will hear a chorus of ohhs and ahhs! Don't forget the large green salad!

Rip's Sedona retreat was a life-changing experience for us both. We had previously read Rip's books and attended his weekend introductory seminar. However, it wasn't until we experienced this week of camaraderie and foodie experiences, particularly with Jane and Ann, that it became clear to us that our dramatic change in diet is so overwhelmingly supported by an ability to simply and effectively prepare food that is as delicious as it is nutritional.

Our doctor could hardly believe the almost immediate and dramatic effect on our health metrics. We're both convinced we will enjoy many "extra" years of feeling and looking great with our children and grandchildren.

—Carl Acebes, age 70, and Carol Acebes, age 70,
Acebes Family Office

Rescue Family Suppers

Rib-Stickin' Burrito

Burritos, burritos, burritos. They are the small burros that carry heavy loads. That is how burritos got their name. We want you to pack the rice, beans, chiles, peppers, corn, cilantro, onions, and all the other leftovers from the night before into a wrap and roll it up—like a donkey carrying a load. That'll do, Burrito!

Makes 6 burritos

INGREDIENTS:

½ cup brown rice
1 onion, diced
4 ounces mushrooms, sliced
1 clove garlic, minced
1 red bell pepper, diced
4 ounces fresh spinach
1 (15-ounce) can fat-free vegetarian refried beans
1 (15-ounce) can black beans, drained and rinsed

½ cup salsa
1 teaspoon ground cumin
½ teaspoon garlic powder
Pinch of cayenne pepper
6 whole-grain wraps or tortillas or Lavash brand bread, no added oil (heat these up a bit if they are not flexible)

OPTIONAL TOPPINGS:

Romaine lettuce, chopped
Cherry tomatoes, halved
Jicama, shredded

Fresh cilantro, chopped
Hot sauce

INSTRUCTIONS:

Prepare the rice per package instructions. Set aside.

Preheat the oven to 350°F. Line a baking sheet with parchment paper or use a nonstick baking sheet. In a large pan over high heat, cook the onion, mushrooms, garlic, red pepper, and spinach until tender. Decrease the heat to medium and add the refried beans, black beans, and brown rice; stir well to combine. Add your favorite salsa, cumin, garlic powder, and cayenne and stir until the mixture is evenly mixed.

Make sure the wraps are warm and flexible before building the burritos or they will crack. Scoop ½ cup or more of the mixture into the center area of a burrito wrap. Fold over the sides and place the burrito on the lined baking sheet—use metal utensils to hold the sides down if they unfold. Continue assembling the burritos and placing them side by side on the baking sheet.

For crispy burritos, bake uncovered; for softer burritos, cover with aluminum foil. Bake for 12 to 15 minutes, or until warmed and browned to your liking. Serve with your favorite salsa and other optional toppings like romaine, cherry tomatoes, shredded jicama, chopped cilantro, and hot sauce—alongside a heaping green salad.

Sloppy Joe Tostados

This is a piled-high, sloppy, crispy mountain of familiar flavor, mess, and fun.

Serves 4

INGREDIENTS:

8 corn tortillas
2 (15-ounce) cans prepared brown lentils (or 1½ cups dry lentils)
1 medium onion, diced
1 green bell pepper, diced
4 ounces (about 1 cup) mushrooms, sliced
6 ounces tomato paste
1 (15-ounce) can diced tomatoes, drained
4 tablespoons barbecue sauce (we prefer Bone Suckin' Sauce)
2 teaspoons chili powder
¼ teaspoon smoked paprika
1 teaspoon pure maple syrup

INSTRUCTIONS:

Preheat the oven to 350°F.

Place the corn tortillas flat and directly on the oven rack. Check the tortillas after 8 minutes. If they are dry and hard, they are ready. If not, leave them in, checking every 2 minutes to see if they are dry and hard. Once they cool they get crispy. That is when we call them tostados!

If starting with dry lentils, combine 1½ cups dry lentils and 3½ cups water in a pot. Bring to a boil, turn the heat down, and simmer for about 20 minutes, or until the lentils are soft. Drain off any extra water.

In a frying pan over medium heat, cook the onion, pepper, and mushrooms until soft and slightly browned. Add the tomato paste and diced tomatoes and continue to stir over low heat. Add the cooked lentils, barbecue sauce, chili powder, smoked paprika, and maple syrup and thoroughly mix. Reduce the heat to simmer and cook for 5 more minutes.

Taste and tweak the mixture to your liking: Add more maple syrup or barbecue sauce for a sweeter, smokier, or more fiery flavor. Generously spoon the mixture onto your crispy tostados and feast!

Smoky Quinoa Bean Burgers

These burgers are packed with scrumptious ingredients and a mix of flavors that will make this a go-to for lunch or dinner! Try these topped with Roasted Red Peppers (page 266) and other fixings so that they are so tall, you have to eat one open-faced in order to fit your mouth around it!

Makes 4 to 6 burgers

INGREDIENTS:

1 onion, diced
½ cup cooked quinoa
1 (15-ounce) can black beans, drained and rinsed
1 (15-ounce) can cannellini beans, drained and rinsed
2 tablespoons low-sodium tamari
2 cloves garlic, minced
½ cup packed cilantro sprigs
1 teaspoon ground cumin
¼ teaspoon cayenne pepper
¼ teaspoon smoked paprika

½ cup chickpea flour (aka garbanzo bean flour)
½ to ¾ cup whole wheat panko (aka bread crumbs: we prefer Ian's brand; for gluten-free, use corn-based crumbs)
Pinch of black pepper
4 whole-grain burger buns (for gluten-free, order Millet and Flax Hamburger Buns from www.samisbakery.com)

TOPPINGS, YOUR CHOICE:

Arugula
Ketchup
Mustard
Onion slices

Relish
Spinach
Tomato slices

INSTRUCTIONS:

Line a baking sheet with parchment paper.

In a frying pan over high heat, cook the onion while stirring constantly and slowly reducing the heat until it begins to brown and soften, 5 to 6 minutes.

Place the onion, cooked quinoa, black beans, cannellini beans, tamari, garlic, cilantro, cumin, cayenne, and smoked paprika in a food processor and blend until a finely chopped mixture forms.

Transfer the mixture to a medium bowl and add the flour, ½ cup of the panko, and a pinch of black pepper. If the mixture is too loose to hold its form, stir in the rest of the panko.

Using a ½-cup measure, form the mixture into round balls, then gently press them into patties on the parchment-lined pan. Once all the patties are formed, cover and chill until firm, at least 20 minutes.

Preheat the oven to 375°F. Bake the burgers for 20 to 25 minutes, or until golden brown.

Place the burgers on a platter and serve on open-faced whole-grain buns with all the toppings you love!

Grandpa's Homemade Eat Loaf

This plant-strong loaf of love tastes just like a visit to Grandma and Grandpa's house. These familiar flavors warm the soul... especially now that we know the original recipe is no longer clogging our hearts!

Serves 4

INGREDIENTS:

1 large onion, minced
1 teaspoon minced garlic
1 red bell pepper, minced
4 ounces mushrooms, sliced
¼ cup shredded or chopped carrots
1 (15-ounce) can kidney beans, drained and rinsed
1 (15-ounce) can cannellini beans, drained and rinsed
1 cup old-fashioned oats
½ cup nutritional yeast
2 teaspoons low-sodium tamari
1 teaspoon paprika
½ teaspoon black pepper
1 teaspoon dried rosemary
½ teaspoon onion powder
½ teaspoon dry mustard
1 teaspoon ground sage
¼ to ½ cup barbecue sauce (we prefer Bone Suckin' Sauce) or ketchup

INSTRUCTIONS:

Preheat the oven to 350°F.

In a nonstick frying pan, cook the onion for a few minutes on medium-high heat until it begins to soften. Add the garlic, red pepper, mushrooms, and carrots and continue cooking for 5 to 8 minutes, or until the mushrooms are soft.

In a medium bowl, mix together the kidney beans, cannellini beans, oats, nutritional yeast, tamari, paprika, black pepper, rosemary, onion powder, dry mustard, and sage. Add the cooked vegetable mixture to the bowl and stir. Use your hands here to mix, mash, and squish most of the beans. When it becomes sort of sticky, it is ready for the loaf pan.

Coat the bottom of a loaf pan with ¼ cup (or less) of barbecue sauce and add the vegetable and bean mixture. Try to level the surface before spreading another thick layer of barbecue sauce on top.

Bake for 1 hour. Allow this dish to cool a bit. It cuts MUCH better when it has had time to cool and set.

Serve warm with a pile of cooked greens or a large green salad!

Triple Pepper Chipotle Chili

This blue-ribbon chili recipe serves eight or more, so call up family and friends to share this champion of yum! The trick is soaking the chipotle pepper the night before. Jane loves it because she can wake up in the morning with a dinner plan in place!

Serves 8

INGREDIENTS:

- ½ to 1 chipotle pepper, dried (not soaked in adobo sauce)
- 2 cups brown rice
- 1 large onion, julienned
- 1 red bell pepper, diced
- 1 orange bell pepper, diced
- 1 green bell pepper, diced
- 4 celery stalks, sliced
- 1 medium zucchini, diced
- 8 ounces mushrooms, sliced
- 1 cup carrots, julienned or matchstick
- 2 (28-ounce) cans peeled whole tomatoes, with their juices
- 5 tablespoons chili powder
- 1 teaspoon ground cumin
- 2 (15-ounce) cans kidney beans, drained and rinsed
- ½ cup barbecue sauce
- 2 tablespoons pure maple syrup
- ½ cup salsa

INSTRUCTIONS:

In a small bowl, place the dried chipotle pepper, cover with water, and let soak overnight.

The next day, prepare the rice per package directions. Set aside.

In a pot over medium-high heat, simmer together the onion, the bell peppers, celery, zucchini, mushrooms, and carrots for about 10 minutes, or until the onions are translucent, the carrots are tender but not soft, and the mushrooms are cooked through.

Decrease the heat to low. Add the tomatoes and their juice. Once in the pot, cut the whole tomatoes into pieces using the edge of a spoon, a knife, or kitchen scissors. Add the chili powder and cumin.

Finely mince the soaked chipotle pepper and add the desired amount to the pot along with the kidney beans, your favorite barbecue sauce, maple syrup, and salsa of your choice;stir together for a minute or two.

Simmer on low for 30 minutes. Add extra salsa, maple syrup, chili powder, or chipotle pepper to your taste. Keep warm until ready to serve. Line the serving bowls with brown rice, heap on the chili, and don't forget your green salad!

The Launcher Quesadilla

This recipe is called the Launcher because once people try these quesadillas they are ready to launch into the lifestyle— no more questions asked. One of our close friends tried to get her family plant-based with all sorts of recipes—nothing worked, not one thing. Then she served them these quesadillas, and they climbed aboard!

Makes two 9-inch-diameter quesadillas

INGREDIENTS:

1 medium sweet potato
½ cup cooked brown rice
½ cup salsa, plus more for serving
½ red bell pepper, diced
1 (15-ounce) can black beans, drained and rinsed
¼ teaspoon onion powder
¼ teaspoon chili powder
¼ teaspoon ground cumin
½ cup fresh spinach
3 to 4 whole wheat tortillas, or rice or corn tortillas (with no added oil)
½ fresh jalapeño pepper, minced (optional)
Hot sauce, for serving

INSTRUCTIONS:

Prepare the sweet potato any way you prefer:

Microwave a whole sweet potato for about 8 minutes, or until soft. Remove and discard the skin from the orange flesh. Set aside.

Or, preheat the oven to 400°F. Line a baking sheet with parchment paper and bake the sweet potato on the lined pan in the oven for 45 minutes to 1 hour, or until soft. Skin removal optional.

Or, peel the sweet potato, cube it, and place in a steamer basket. Place at least 2 inches of water in the bottom of the steamer, cover, and steam for 8 to 10 minutes, or until soft.

Transfer the sweet potato to a mixing bowl and mash until smooth—similar to the texture of baby food. To the bowl add the cooked rice, salsa, pepper, black beans, onion powder, chili powder, and cumin to taste; stir to incorporate. Add the spinach and stir again.

Place a tortilla in a nonstick frying pan over medium heat and slather with the sweet potato–bean mixture. Add minced jalapeño, if using.

Place a second tortilla on top of the first. Press down on the top tortilla with a spatula, then cook in the pan for about 3 minutes, or until the filling is warm and the tortilla browns a bit. Flip with a spatula and cook the opposite side for 3 minutes more, or until cooked to your liking. Transfer the quesadilla to a cutting board and divide into the desired number of sections. Serve topped with your favorite salsa and hot sauce.

BBQ Bellas and Other Fellas

The only thing better than the smell of these portabellas cooking and their magnetic visual appeal is stepping up and sinking your teeth into this burst of BBQ'd goodness.

Serves 2 to 4

INGREDIENTS:

4 portabella mushroom caps
1 large onion, sliced into
   1-inch-square chunks
8 ounces mushrooms, sliced
½ to 1 cup barbecue sauce (we
   prefer Bone Suckin' Sauce)

4 to 6 cups kale or any greens,
   leaves stripped from spines
   and torn into bite-size pieces
4 cups cooked brown rice

INSTRUCTIONS:

Preheat the oven to 350°F.

Line a baking sheet or lasagna-size baking dish with parchment paper.

Trim the stems off the portabella caps. Place the portabella caps, onion, and sliced mushrooms in the lined pan; include the stems if you are so inclined. Arrange the portabella mushrooms so they are gill side up. Spread barbecue sauce over the gills; drizzle it over the onion chunks and mushroom slices as well. Bake for 40 minutes.

In a frying pan or pot, place the kale in 2 inches of boiling water, cover, and cook for 4 to 6 minutes, or until the preferred tenderness is reached. Drain well.

In each bowl, place a layer of warm rice, then a layer of kale, and top with mushrooms and onions. Serve with a large green salad!

Quinoa Cali Rolls

Jane's friend Eleanor Rimmerman tested this recipe on her cardiologist father, and he told her that he could eat the whole dish by himself! We love it! And, we hope these rolls are part of his marching orders for patients going forward. These are especially fun to make with a group of friends.

Makes about 7 rolls

INGREDIENTS:

1 cup red quinoa
1 cup short grain brown rice
2 tablespoons brown rice vinegar, if needed
1 package nori sheets (usually contains 7 to 10 sheets)
1 red bell pepper, seeded and julienned
4 scallions, chopped

½ cucumber, peeled, seeded, and cut lengthwise into thin strips
2 carrots, shredded
1 mango, peeled, and cut into strips (optional—but we love this!)
8 spears asparagus, steamed
Wasabi powder
Pickled ginger
Low-sodium tamari

INSTRUCTIONS:

Prepare the red quinoa and brown rice per the package directions.

Place the cooked quinoa and cooked brown rice in a large bowl. Stir them together until they become sort of sticky—to the point where the mixture holds onto the spoon. (Note: If the rice is not sticking to the quinoa, stir in the brown rice vinegar until the texture becomes sticky.)

Place one sheet of nori flat on a dry surface. Spread about ½ cup quinoa and rice on one-half of the flat sheet.

Place the vegetables of your choice horizontally in the middle of the flattened quinoa and rice. Using both hands, starting from the end covered with quinoa and rice, roll up the sheet. Carefully cover the vegetables and keep rolling. The roll will stick to itself especially well if the quinoa and rice are still a little warm. If your nori does not stick, try dabbing the edge of the non-rice-covered end with water.

Slice each roll with a sharp knife into ½-inch, medallion-style pieces.

Make the desired amount of wasabi paste by adding water to the wasabi powder as directed.

Serve the nori pieces with little dishes of pickled ginger, wasabi, and low-sodium tamari. Dip each nori roll into the wasabi and tamari and top with ginger as desired. Or you can eat them just as they are along with a huge green salad or a pile of cooked greens.

Lazy Days Tostados

Of all the wonderful combinations of various foods people have devised over the centuries, beans and potatoes have to be one of the most earthy, satisfying, and delicious. Enjoy a lovely, lazy day and this perfect ancient combo.

Serves 2

INGREDIENTS:

2 Yukon Gold potatoes
1 (8-ounce) can black beans, drained and rinsed
1 (8-ounce) can refried pinto beans, vegetarian with no added oil or sugar (we recommend Casa Fiesta brand)

½ teaspoon ground cumin
½ teaspoon chili powder
¼ teaspoon garlic powder
4 to 6 corn tortillas (no oil added!)
Salsa
Fresh cilantro, for garnish
2 green onions, chopped, for garnish

INSTRUCTIONS:

Preheat the oven to 400°F.

Bake the potatoes in the oven for about 40 minutes, or until cooked through. Allow them to cool for 5 to 10 minutes, then place in a bowl. With a fork or potato masher, smash the potatoes so they are chunky yet stick together. Set aside the warm semi-smashed potatoes.

In a pot over medium heat, cook the black beans and refried beans for 5 minutes, or until warm. With the back of a spoon, smash about half of the whole beans right in the pot. This creates a thicker, creamier bean texture. Add the cumin, chili powder, and garlic powder. Stir well and taste, adjusting seasoning as desired. Set aside.

In a frying pan over low heat, arrange as many tortillas as will fit flat. Warm them until soft and flexible. Place 1 or 2 tortillas on each plate. On top of each tortilla, place a layer of potatoes and a layer of beans. Top with your salsa of choice, add a garnish of cilantro and green onion, and eat immediately. Serve along with a huge green salad or a pile of cooked greens.

Portabella Fajitas

Thank goodness for the versatile portabella mushroom. It can be dressed up or down for a fine dinner date or a quick on-the-go lunch. This recipe is somewhere in between!

Serves 4

INGREDIENTS:

½ cup brown rice, uncooked
1 to 2 tablespoons Fajita Seasoning (page 263)
1 onion, sliced into strips
1 red bell pepper, sliced into thick strips
1 green bell pepper, sliced into thick strips
2 portabella caps, sliced into thick strips
6 corn tortillas
2 green onions, chopped, for garnish
1 avocado, sliced or mashed (allow ¼ avocado maximum per serving)

INSTRUCTIONS:

Prepare the rice per package instructions. Set aside.

Prepare the fajita seasoning.

In a frying pan over high heat (so hot that a bead of water does not turn to steam but rolls around on the surface), add the sliced onion strips. Stir the onions, allowing them to brown, for about 3 minutes.

Reduce the heat to medium-high. Add the red pepper and green pepper strips and cook, stirring constantly, for about 3 more minutes.

Add the mushroom strips to the pan and allow them to cook, stirring constantly, for 3 to 5 more minutes. Taste a mushroom to make sure it is cooked all the way through. Turn the heat down to medium. Add 1 tablespoon of fajita seasoning or more to taste.

Warm the corn tortillas (so they are flexible and don't crack when used) by either wrapping in foil and heating in a 300°F oven for 5 to 10 minutes or placing in a dry frying pan over medium-low heat and flipping to warm both sides.

In the center fold of a warmed corn tortilla, press about ¼ cup of brown rice, then a layer of fajita-seasoned portabellas and veggies. Fold the side over, garnish with green onions and avocado, and serve alongside a huge green salad or a pile of cooked greens.

Easy No-Recipe Meal Ideas

Throngs of people, from firefighters to parents to pilot study participants, have written us to say they have become Engine 2 experts at making superfast nutritious meals. Following are some of their favorite combinations of ingredients. Play around with these simple no-recipe recipe ideas and open your eyes and mouths to the infinite combinations sitting in your fridge, freezer, and pantry, all at the ends of your fingertips!

(Tip: For even faster meal prep, use frozen veggies, rice, potatoes, or quinoa.)

Suggested no-recipe meal ingredients:

Kale, brown rice, black beans, ¼ avocado, hot sauce

Whole-grain pasta, diced tomatoes, basil, mushrooms, garlic

Brown rice, chickpeas, pineapple, green onions, barbecue sauce

Quinoa, kidney beans, lime juice, oregano, cucumber, arugula

Sweet potato, kale, white beans, brown rice

Engine 2 Crispbread, oil-free hummus, tomato slices, fresh basil

White potato, black beans, tomatoes, corn, spinach, cumin

Quinoa, mixed greens, red beans, cauliflower, basil

Brown rice, kidney beans, diced tomatoes, zucchini, garlic, oregano

White beans, fingerling potatoes, Brussels sprouts, garlic

Roasted vegetable mix, quinoa, garlic and herb blend salt-free seasoning

Cauliflower, chickpeas, potatoes, curry powder, onions, brown rice

Lentils, collard greens, brown rice, salt-free mesquite seasoning

Potatoes, portabella mushrooms, green beans, spinach, black beans

Salad greens, lentils, cherry tomatoes, red onions, oil-free salad dressing

Engine 2 Whole-Grain Pizza Crust, mushrooms, spinach, onions, oil-free pasta sauce

Brown rice, salsa, frozen Southwestern veggie mix, black beans

Mushrooms, crushed tomatoes, onions, whole-grain macaroni, lentils, garlic, oregano, basil

Salad topped with roasted potato wedges, black beans, hummus, and salsa

Whole-grain tortilla, oil-free hummus, cucumbers, mixed greens, tomatoes

Whole-grain pasta, zucchini, broccoli, peppers, onions, mushrooms, tomatoes

Salad of chopped cucumber, celery, carrots, and zucchini, tossed with quinoa

Grilled zucchini and mushrooms with oil-free hummus on whole-grain bread

Roasted potato wedges (oil-free), Engine 2 Plant-Strong Burgers, and a big salad with oil-free dressing

Whole-grain pasta cooked and chilled, cucumber, tomato, beans, balsamic vinegar

Lentils, chopped tomato, lettuce, spinach, and salsa, served on lettuce or served in corn tortillas

Diced potatoes, pinto beans, onions, peppers, spinach, black pepper, garlic

Butternut squash, lentils, and salt-free Southwestern seasoning, over red rice with steamed kale

Mashed chickpeas, onion, garlic, chopped celery, and cucumber served on whole-grain bread

Stuffed ancient grains wrap: hummus, onions, tomatoes, mixed greens, cucumber, sprouts

Quinoa, pineapple, cilantro, onion, kale, chipotle, chili sauce

Sweet potato topped with black beans, cilantro, and salsa

Wild rice, onion, lentils, greens, and salt-free seasoning of your choice

Brown rice, black pepper, Asian-style veggie mix

Engine 2 Grain Medleys Morning Blend topped with fresh fruit

Steamed potatoes, lentils with barbecue sauce, steamed green beans

Mixing Bowl Salad: loaded up with greens, veggies, beans, balsamic vinegar

Ezekiel 4:9 Bread, Engine 2 Burger, tomato slices, barbecue sauce, and a side of greens

Whole-grain pasta, black beans, corn, peppers, nutritional yeast, cumin, cilantro

Mashed sweet potatoes, pinto beans with barbecue sauce, steamed collard greens

Brown rice, diced green onions, broccoli, diced carrots, lemon juice, black pepper

Black beans, green peppers, onions, diced tomatoes, cumin, chili

DRESSINGS, HUMMUS, TOPPINGS, AND SIDES

What in the world are you going to put on your world-class salads? Why, one of these robust and delicious salad dressings, of course! Each one has a unique flavor profile. Play with all of them over the course of the Seven-Day Rescue and see which one steals the show!

Amazon Salad Dressing

This is a gem from the jungle—it adds swing to any salad.

Makes about 1 cup

INGREDIENTS:

3 tablespoons lime juice
½ teaspoon ground cumin
2 green onions, chopped
2 tablespoons chopped fresh cilantro or basil

1 tablespoon minced fresh jalapeño pepper
1 mango, peeled and cubed

INSTRUCTIONS:

In a food processor or blender, combine the lime juice, cumin, green onion, cilantro, jalapeño, and mango. Blend until smooth and serve.

Sesame Seed Dressing

This is one well-rounded dressing: nutty, sweet, salty, and smart.

Makes about ½ cup

INGREDIENTS:

3 tablespoons sesame seeds, home-toasted
2 tablespoons maple syrup

2 tablespoons tamari

INSTRUCTIONS:

In a frying pan over medium-low heat, toast the sesame seeds. Watch the seeds closely, stirring occasionally, and toast until the seeds are browned and fragrant. In a bowl, whisk the ingredients together, adding water to achieve the desired texture, and serve.

Sweet Fire Dressing

You will love the delicate balance of flavor and heat in this dressing! This is one fire Rip doesn't have to put out.

Makes 1 cup

INGREDIENTS:

½ cup plain oat milk
½ teaspoon cayenne pepper
⅛ teaspoon smoked paprika

¼ cup Dijon mustard or spicy
   brown mustard
¼ cup pure maple syrup

INSTRUCTIONS:

Combine the oat milk, cayenne, paprika, mustard, and maple syrup in a bowl; stir well and serve.

Ginger Miso Dressing

You may want to have this fresh ginger and miso blend every single day of the week. If you are lucky enough to have any left over, try it as a sauce when you build your own Rescue Supper Bowl (pages 232–243)!

Makes about ½ cup

INGREDIENTS:

2 tablespoons white miso
2 teaspoons peeled and grated
   fresh ginger
2 tablespoons pure maple syrup

1 tablespoon rice vinegar
3 tablespoons water
1 teaspoon sesame seeds

INSTRUCTIONS:

Whisk together all of the ingredients. Serve over a green salad or cooked greens.

Jane's Dancing Dressing

3-2-1! It's easy because those three numbers are the amounts of the ingredients. Jane says, "Go ahead, give this dressing a go. I bet you will keep dancing right back to it!"

Makes about ½ cup

INGREDIENTS:

3 tablespoons balsamic vinegar
2 tablespoons mustard
1 tablespoon pure maple syrup

1 tablespoon fresh lemon juice
Chopped fresh dill (optional)

INSTRUCTIONS:

Combine the vinegar, mustard, maple syrup, and lemon juice in a bowl and whisk until uniformly mixed. Add the chopped fresh dill, if using. Serve over a green salad or cooked greens.

Ann and Essy's Favorite

This dressing is a given every single night for our parents, Ann and Essy. Maybe, just maybe, this will become your constant dinner companion, too!

Makes ½ cup

INGREDIENTS:

2 tablespoons Our Hummus (page 260) or hummus made with no tahini or oil added
2 tablespoons orange juice, or sections and juice of ½ orange

2 tablespoons balsamic vinegar
2 teaspoons mustard
1 teaspoon minced fresh ginger

INSTRUCTIONS:

In a small bowl, mix the hummus, orange juice, balsamic vinegar, your favorite mustard, and the ginger together with a fork. Toss with a green salad and enjoy.

Walnut Garlic Dressing

This is a creamy-dreamy delight that has dressed the Esselstyn family salads and leafy greens for decades.

Makes ¾ cup

INGREDIENTS:

⅓ cup walnuts
⅓ cup chickpeas
1 tablespoon low-sodium tamari

1 clove garlic
⅓ cup plus 2 tablespoons water

INSTRUCTIONS:

In a food processor or high-speed blender, combine the walnuts, chickpeas, tamari, garlic, and water. When creamy and well combined, it's ready to serve!

Hummus

Hummus is your new best friend, your new go-to spread, your new cheese, your new mayo, butter, and oil. Yup, hummus. It is your new base for salad dressings, spreads for sandwiches, or dips for your cocktail party. The Hummuses are here!

Our Hummus

Note: Our Hummus has a mustard kick, so if you are not a mustard fan, reduce the amount of brown mustard. Also, if you are low on chickpeas, try cannellini beans!

Makes 1¼ cups

INGREDIENTS:

1 (15-ounce) can chickpeas, no
salt, drained and well rinsed
2 large cloves garlic
2 tablespoons lemon juice
2 tablespoons water

Black pepper
1½ tablespoons brown mustard
¼ teaspoon salt (optional; we do
not use it)

INSTRUCTIONS:

Mix the chickpeas, garlic, lemon juice, water, pepper to taste, mustard, and salt, if using, in a food processor until uniformly smooth.

Serve immediately; refrigerate the extra.

Black Bean Hummus

Jane's husband, Brian, knows his way around the kitchen. His black bean hummus is exactly what it should be: flavorful, smooth, and well rounded. Brian knows how to do it, like an artist who sketches without hesitation.

Makes 1½ cups

INGREDIENTS:

1 (15-ounce) can black beans, drained and rinsed
1 teaspoon Dijon mustard
1 teaspoon ground cumin
1 clove garlic

2 tablespoons salsa
1 teaspoon orange juice
Sriracha or other hot sauce of your choice

INSTRUCTIONS:

In a food processor, combine the beans, mustard, cumin, garlic, salsa, and orange juice and blend. Add water as needed to reach the desired texture. Add sriracha to taste.

Red Pepper Hummus

This hummus is versatile—eat it with veggies, make a sandwich (see the Red Pepper Smile Flat on page 222), use it as a salad dressing substitute, or, as the recipe inventor, Eleanor Rimmerman, discovered, add a bit of water and make a tasty pasta sauce. This hummus adds a pop of color, and it's downright cool across the board.

Makes 1½ to 2 cups

INGREDIENTS:

1 (15-ounce) can cannellini beans, drained and rinsed
1 large clove garlic, minced
2 tablespoons fresh-squeezed lemon juice

1 small red bell pepper, seeds and stems removed, chopped; or ½ cup Roasted Red Peppers (page 266)
¼ teaspoon salt (optional)

INSTRUCTIONS:

In a food processor, combine the cannellini beans, garlic, lemon juice, red pepper, and salt, if using, Blend until uniformly smooth or to desired consistency. If the hummus is too runny, add a few additional tablespoons of cannellini beans. If it is too thick, add more red pepper.

Sweet Potato Convert Hummus

The Cleveland Clinic Wellness Institute chef, Jim Perko, created this creamy, flavorful, and beautiful hummus that can make a plant-based convert out of anyone!

Makes 2 cups

INGREDIENTS:

1 large sweet potato, baked and peeled

1 large red bell pepper, roasted, seeded, and skin removed; or 1 (4-ounce) jar roasted red peppers, drained and blackened skin removed

3 tablespoons lemon juice

1 clove garlic, minced

½ teaspoon ground cumin

Pinch of cayenne pepper

1 tablespoon fresh parsley (whichever kind you like), chopped

INSTRUCTIONS:

In a food processor, combine the sweet potato, red pepper, lemon juice, garlic, cumin, and cayenne.

Process until the mixture is smooth. Transfer to a serving bowl and refrigerate for at least 1 hour. Sprinkle with chopped parsley before serving.

Quick Blueberry Topping

Jane's house is filled with picky teenagers who are especially so with fruit. "Growl," is what Jane used to say. Now she says, "Let's make Quick Blueberry Topping." This is a yummy blueberry sauce (some call it a coulis), which we all love on Oat Waffles (page 206), Oat Pancakes (page 205), or any of our oatmeals.

Makes 1+ cups

INGREDIENTS:

1½ cups blueberries (in our house we use the ones that are too soft for the kids' liking)

Juice of 2 clementines or 1 orange

INSTRUCTIONS:

In a small pot over medium heat, combine the blueberries and the juice from the clementines—we use a lemon press or a citrus reamer to get the juice out—and bring to a boil. Turn the heat down to a simmer for 5 to 10 minutes, or until the mixture becomes syrup-like. If you like the texture of the topping at this stage, serve it up now. If you want it smoother, pour the sauce into a blender or food processor and blend until the mixture is appropriately smooth.

Serve and enjoy, or place in an airtight container and refrigerate.

Fajita Seasoning

This seasoning adds flavor to your Portabella Fajitas (page 253) or any other dish you think needs a little cha-cha-cha! Make a jar of this seasoning for the week.

Makes about ¼ cup

INGREDIENTS:

2 teaspoons chili powder
1 teaspoon paprika
½ teaspoon onion powder
½ teaspoon garlic powder

½ teaspoon ground cumin
¼ teaspoon cayenne pepper
¼ teaspoon oregano
Pinch of salt (optional)

INSTRUCTIONS:

In a small-lidded container or jar, combine the chili powder, paprika, onion powder, garlic powder, cumin, cayenne, oregano, and salt, if using. Shake well.

Cooked Kale

There are as many ways to eat kale, collards, and other greens as there are people who eat them. Try kale with a variety of infused balsamic vinegars or plant-strong dressings—you'll find one that works for you and become best friends! Or maybe you'll become best friends with them all! It doesn't matter as long as you add kale or another leafy green into your body and into your day.

Serves 6

INGREDIENTS:

2 bunches kale, leaves stripped from the spines and torn into bite-size pieces

INSTRUCTIONS:

Place kale in a large pot of boiling water, cover, and cook about 5 minutes, or to desired tenderness, and drain in a colander.

Cooked Onions

Almost every cooked meal starts with an onion. This step can trip some people up, since it is a knee-jerk response to add oil to the pan. Read my lips...No oil is needed! It doesn't matter what sort of pan you use. You'll learn to love cooking onions without oil as they turn brown and caramelize. Give it a try—all you need is heat and a pan.

Makes 1½ to 2 cups

INGREDIENTS:

1 large onion, diced or julienned

INSTRUCTIONS:

Place a frying pan over high heat. Wait until the pan is so hot that a drop of water does not turn to steam when dropped into the pan, but rather beads around like a pearl on the surface.

When it is that hot, add the onion and stir until it starts to brown.

As you stir, slowly reduce the heat and continue cooking the onion. Add a teaspoon of water and continue stirring until the onion is browned and cooked through.

Serve warm or store covered in the fridge until ready to use.

Cooked Mushrooms

Mushrooms bring a sink-your-teeth-into-my-fungi sort of texture and a satisfying umami flavor that together make a recipe rock!

Makes ½ cup

INGREDIENTS:

8 ounces mushrooms, sliced

INSTRUCTIONS:

Place a frying pan over high heat. Place the sliced mushrooms flat in the pan. No mushroom should be resting on any other mushroom—all flat surfaces in contact with the heated pan. Let them cook for a few minutes. Really. Let them be. In a few minutes you will see them starting to brown and become fragrant.

After 4 to 5 minutes, turn them over and brown the other side.

Add a little water if needed; otherwise, stir them around in their own juices and cook for 2 more minutes. Serve warm or store covered in the fridge until ready to use.

Cooked Broccoli

Rip's neighbor, Blake Trabulsi, makes the best broccoli ever! Rip's kids Kole and Sophie always come home after eating some of their broccoli for dinner and ask why they can't have broccoli like Blake's! So, Rip asked Blake what his trick was for making perfect broccoli, and with a devilish grin he replied that it's all about the timing, the color, and the magic of the fork. Read on! His trick is wickedly simple, as you shall see.

Makes about 2 cups

INGREDIENTS:

2 broccoli crowns, broken into florets (about 2 cups)

INSTRUCTIONS:

Fill a pot with about 2 inches of water. Place the broccoli florets in the steamer basket, place it in the pot, and turn the heat to high and cover. (Set a timer for 10 minutes once you light the fire if you have a gas stove.) The trick here is not to overcook the broccoli. It is done when the color is a bright brilliant green and you can stick a fork into the stalk fairly easily. Take the broccoli out at 10 minutes and immediately dump on a plate—that's the trick! Do not let the broccoli sit in a covered pot. Get it on a plate quickly.

Our mom, Ann, encourages all the grandchildren to eat their vegetables plain in order to learn to like the actual flavor of the food. So try it! Serve the brilliant broccoli plain, or sprinkle with a little bit of seasoning or spices of your choice.

Roasted Red Peppers

Rip can stand over the sink and eat these all day long! The flavor and texture are devilishly good. We add these to salads, salad dressings, sandwiches, wraps, rice, grains, greens, burgers, beans—anything! Wow yourself and others with these flavorful and savory strips!

Makes 1½ to 2 cups

INGREDIENTS:

3 red peppers
1½ tablespoons balsamic vinegar
1 teaspoon minced garlic
½ teaspoon dried basil
½ teaspoon dried thyme

1 teaspoon Italian seasoning (or
    ½ teaspoon dried rosemary,
    ½ teaspoon dried marjoram,
    and ½ teaspoon dried oregano)

INSTRUCTIONS:

Preheat the oven to 450°F or broil. Place the peppers on a baking sheet and roast until blackened on one side, then continue rotating the peppers until all sides are blackened, about 8 minutes per side, or until the peppers start to collapse. Some people prefer to roast peppers individually over a gas flame, which also works.

Place the roasted red peppers, no matter your roasting technique, in a paper bag and wrap in a towel for 10 minutes. This allows the skin to lift off the pepper flesh and makes the peeling easier. Remove the peppers from the bag and peel off the skins, saving any resulting juice. Slice or tear the pepper flesh into long strips and place in a bowl, discarding seeds and stems. Add the vinegar, garlic, basil, thyme, and Italian seasoning. Allow the peppers and spices to marinate for at least 30 minutes. Add the juice from the peeling process, if available, to the bowl as well.

Dressings and Topping Tips

Great toppings for salads, greens, and an assortment of dishes abound.

Dressings. Use any dressing in the "Dressings, Hummus, Toppings, and Sides" section over your salads or drizzled on your greens, or dunk your sandwiches in them! These dressings are all clean and fine to use in abundance. They save us from the gallons of oil, dairy, grease, and cheese we used to love before we got a divorce from those bad boys.

Infused Balsamic Vinegars. We used to think of vinegars as used only for dyeing Easter eggs and cleaning floors. Now we see them as irresistible gourmet items. Balsamic vinegars infused with flavors like black currant, lemon, strawberry, mango, maple, and chocolate have invaded our lives and our palates, and we will never turn back. They stand alone as dressings or augment any dish that needs a bit more flavor. Look for fancy vinegar at the grocery and taste-test as many as you can handle! You will be a convert.

Balsamic Glaze. Balsamic glaze is quite sweet and slightly acidic—like a dressing in itself. It costs around $7 or $8, but it's worth every penny because it saves you from the perils of oil-, dairy-, milk-, and cheese-based dressings. We particularly enjoy Cream of Balsamic (deceptively named, since it is dairy-free), made by a company called Isola.

Mustards. Mustard can quiet a palate hungry for texture and depth. It can boost flavor and enhance taste, which makes sandwiches, burgers, or anything else you can imagine more satisfying. We love mustard—it packs a punch and a little goes a long way.

Fruit Topping. A light, sweet, fruit-based topping is a welcome breakfast option for waffles, pancakes, and oatmeal—anything that you might typically pair with maple syrup. See our Quick Blueberry Topping (page 262), or reach for unsweetened applesauce.

Afterword

Thanks for reading this book. I hope you gobbled it all up and are now preparing to set sail on a new adventure in healthy eating and living. You can do this. Don't let anybody or anything get in your way. You deserve it!

I would love to hear about your wonderful successes. Please e-mail me at info@Engine2.com.

All my plant-strong best,
Rip

Appendix 1

Engine 2 Boxed, Packaged, and Canned Approved Shopping List

This is by no means an exhaustive list of all the Engine 2 Seven-Day Rescue–approved products in your local grocery store—but it's a good start. Keep in mind that manufacturers change their ingredients frequently, so please read the label and check the ingredients. Follow the label-reading guidelines in chapter 5, and soon you'll become a seasoned label-reading ninja who can sniff out the good stuff from the bad stuff. Have a blast!

COLD CEREALS (FOUND IN CONVENTIONAL GROCERY STORES)

Arrowhead Mills
> Puffed Corn
> Puffed Kamut
> Puffed Millet
> Puffed Rice
> Puffed Wheat
> Shredded Wheat

Barbara's Bakery
> Shredded Spoonfuls
> Shredded Wheat

Kashi
> Kashi Whole Grain Nuggets
> Kashi Whole Grain Puffs

Nabisco Shredded Wheat
Nature's Path Food
  Corn Puffs
  Kamut Puffs
  Millet Puffs
  Rice Puffs

Post Shredded Wheat
U.S. Mills Uncle Sam Cereal

HOT CEREALS (FOUND IN CONVENTIONAL GROCERY STORES)

Arrowhead Mills
  Bulgar Wheat
  Instant Oatmeal Original
  Oat Bran
  Oat Flakes
  Steel-Cut Oats

Bob's Red Mill
  5, 6, 7, 8, and 10 Grain
  Barley Grits
  Creamy Brown Rice
  Creamy Buckwheat
  Kamut
  Rolled Oats
  Spice N' Nice
  Whole Wheat Farina

McCann's Irish Oatmeal
Quaker Oats
  Barley
  Instant Oatmeal
  Oat Bran

Rolled Oats
Whole Wheat

U.S. Mills
Barley Plus
Brown Rice Cream
Uncle Sam Instant Oatmeal

PASTA AND GRAINS

Continental Mills (à la cracked wheat bulgur)
Eden Quinoa
Fantastic Foods
Brown Basmati Rice
Brown Jasmine Rice

Food Merchants Polenta
Kashi Pilaf
Lundberg Family Farms
Brown Rice
Wild Rice Blends

Quinoa Corp
Quinoa
Quinoa Pasta

San Gennaro Foods Polenta
*Uncle Ben's Instant Brown Rice or Boil-in-Bag Whole Grain
Rice (10-minute cook time)*

Whole wheat pasta is available in most store brands.

Any brown rice, quinoa, or corn pasta is also acceptable (as long as only the single grain is listed in the ingredients). There are also an extraordinary amount of gluten-free pastas out there made from black beans, red lentils, chickpeas, and mung beans, to name just a few.

WHOLE-GRAIN BREADS/TORTILLAS/PIZZA CRUSTS*

Alvarado Street Bakery
Oil-free breads and bagels
Sprouted Wheat Tortillas

Amber Farms
Whole Wheat Pasta Wraps

Bremner Food Group
Natural Ry-Krisp-Fat Free

Brother Juniper's Bakery
100% Whole Wheat
Multigrain

Cedarlane Foods
Fat Free Whole Wheat Tortillas
Whole Wheat Lavash Bread

Dallas Gourmet Bakery
Kabuli Pizza Crust

Food for Life
Ezekiel 4:9 Bread
Sprouted Whole Grain Tortillas

Garden of Eatin'
Bible Bread (regular and salt-free)

Great Harvest Bread Co.
Mestemacher Breads
Rye Bread with Muesli
Natural Rye & Spelt Bread

---

*Since some of these do not meet the 1:1 sodium rule, you should make sure that if your bread is higher in sodium, your entire meal profile is low in sodium and you do not add salt to the overall meal.

Natural Whole Rye Bread
Natural Three Grain Bread

Nature's Hilights, Inc.
Brown Rice Pizza Crust

Nature's Path Foods
Manna Bread

Pure Grain Bakery
Gourmet Rye Bread
Pumpernickel Bread

Ryvita Crispbread
Wasa Crispbread
Hearty
Lite Rye
Multi Grain
Sourdough

Most corn tortillas are also E2-approved.

What to look for at Whole Foods (Whole Foods Brand Foods):

BREADS/TORTILLAS
Engine 2 Tortillas
Brown Rice Tortillas
Sprouted Ancient Grains Tortillas

Engine 2 Crispbreads
Original
Seeds and Spice
Triple Seed

Engine 2 Stone Baked 100% Whole Wheat Pizza Crusts
Engine 2 Sprouted Ancient Grains Burger Buns

Whole Foods 365
Organic Fat-Free Tortillas

BAKED CHIPS
Engine 2 Baked Tortilla Chips
Blue Corn and Black Bean

CANNED BEANS
Whole Foods 365
No-salt-added canned beans
Organic no-salt-added beans
No-salt-added boxed beans

CEREALS
Engine 2 Granola
Apple Pumpkin
Blueberry Vanilla
Plain Jane

Engine 2 Rip's Big Bowl
Banana Walnut
Original
Triple Berry Walnut

Engine 2 Rip's Power Up Bowl
Double Berry (hot cereal)
Original (hot cereal)

Whole Foods 365
Bite-Size Shredded Wheat
Organic Corn Flakes
Organic Multigrain with Flax Instant Oatmeal
Organic Oats and Flax Instant Oatmeal
Organic Old Fashioned Rolled Oats
Organic Original Instant Oatmeal
Organic Quick Oats
Organic Steel Cut Oats

CONDIMENTS

Engine 2 Hummus
- Jalapeño Cilantro
- Roasted Red Pepper
- Spicy Black Bean
- Traditional
- Traditional Snack Pack (three-pack)

Whole Foods 365
- Ketchup
- Reduced Sodium Soy Sauce
- Mustard

NONDAIRY MILK

Engine 2 Almond Milks
- Unsweetened Original
- Unsweetened Vanilla

Pacific Oat Milk
- Original
- Vanilla

Whole Foods 365
- Organic Unsweetened Almond Milk
- Organic Unsweetened Soy Milk

FROZEN FOOD

Engine 2 Grain Medleys
- Ancient Grains Blend
- Fiesta Blend
- Morning Blend
- Wild Rice Blend

Engine 2 Plant-Burger
- Italian Fennel
- Pinto Habanero
- Poblano Black Bean
- Tuscan Kale White Bean

Engine 2 Raviolis
  Chickpea and Spinach
  Butternut Squash and Kale
  Mediterranean Vegetable
  Cannelloni and Kale

Engine 2 Pizzas
  Vegetable Pizza
  BBQ Pizza
  Greens Pizza

Engine 2 Burritos
  Ranchero
  Spicy Green Chili
  Vegetable

Whole Foods 365
  Brown rice
  Frozen fruit (all varieties)
  Frozen vegetables (all varieties)
  Green chickpeas
  Quinoa

PASTA
Whole Foods 365
  Brown Rice
  Whole Wheat Pasta

PASTA SAUCE
Engine 2 Pasta Sauce
  Classic Tomato Basil
  Red Bell Pepper Marinara

SALAD DRESSINGS/DIPS
Health Starts Here Dressings
  Balsamic

Balsamic Fig
Caesar
Garlic Tahini
Sesame Ginger

SALSA

Whole Foods 365
Salsa (look for lowest-sodium options)

SOUPS/BROTHS

Engine 2
Firehouse Chili
Moroccan Style Stew
Vegetable Stock

Appendix 2

Answers to PQ Quiz on Page 33

1. False
2. False
3. True
4. True
5. False
6. False
7. True
8. False
9. True
10. True
11. True
12. False
13. False

Appendix 3

Results from North Ridgeville Seven-Day Pilot Program

What motivated you to join this seven-day study (please select all that apply)?

Answer Options	North Ridgeville
I have a heart disease or had a cardiac event.	2%
I am prediabetic or have type 2 diabetes.	8%
I would like to reduce my medications.	18%
Other (please explain).	18%
I have high blood pressure.	24%
I would like to improve my skin condition.	24%
I have a health concern(s) for a loved one.	26%
I have high cholesterol.	26%
I have arthritic symptoms / joint inflammation.	30%
I am curious to learn more about a plant-based diet.	56%
I have a health concern(s) for myself.	60%
I would like to lose some weight.	84%

Seven-Day Weight-Loss Results (Per Participant)

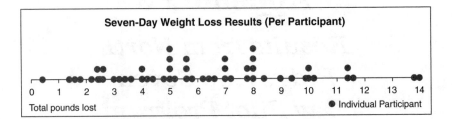

Change in Total Cholesterol in Seven Days

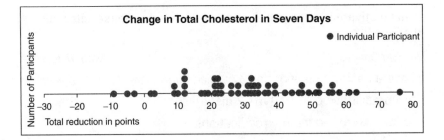

Change in LDL in Seven Days

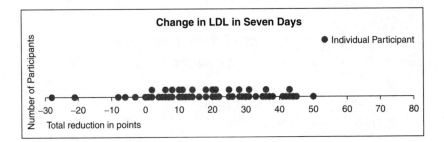

Change in HDL in Seven Days

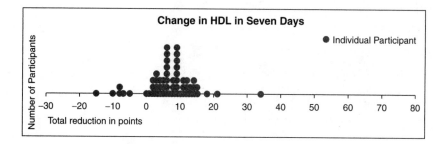

Appendix 4

Nutritional Comparisons

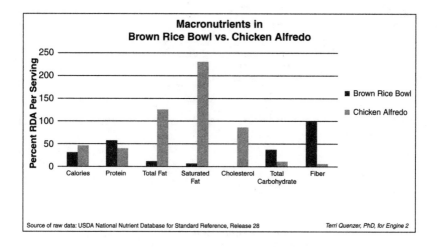

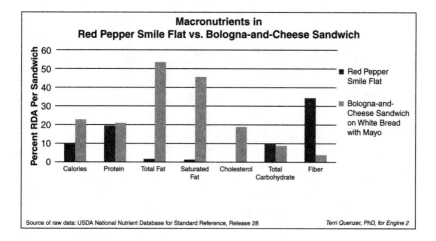

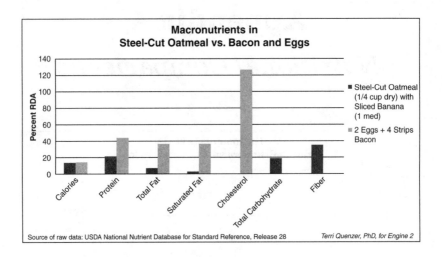

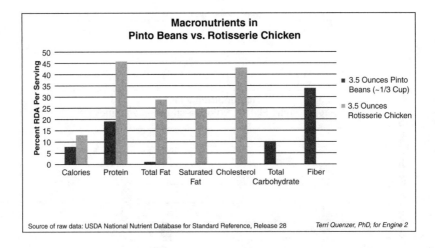

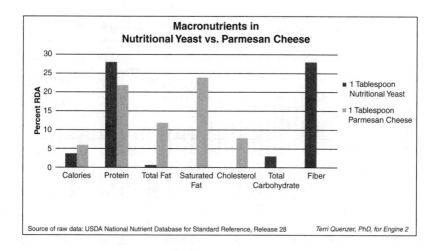

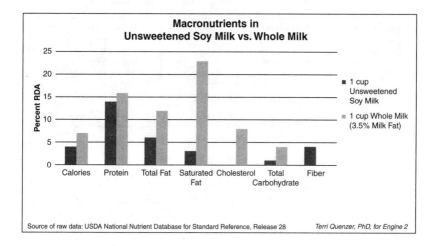

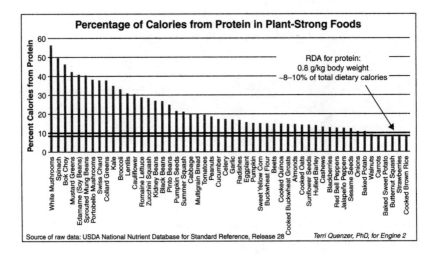

Percentage of Calories from Protein in Plant-Strong Foods

Source of raw data: USDA National Nutrient Database for Standard Reference, Release 28   *Terri Quenzer, PhD, for Engine 2*

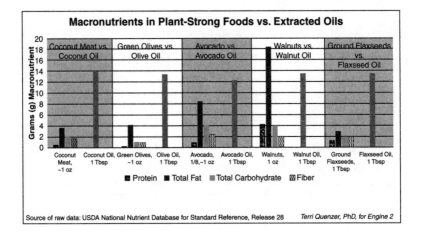

Macronutrients in Plant-Strong Foods vs. Extracted Oils

Source of raw data: USDA National Nutrient Database for Standard Reference, Release 28   *Terri Quenzer, PhD, for Engine 2*

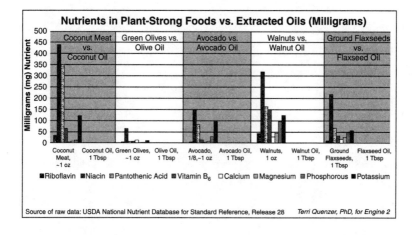

Nutrients in Plant-Strong Foods vs. Extracted Oils (Milligrams)

Source of raw data: USDA National Nutrient Database for Standard Reference, Release 28   *Terri Quenzer, PhD, for Engine 2*

Acknowledgments

First and foremost, I want to thank Whole Foods Market for the opportunity to partner with one of the most extraordinary companies on the planet. In August 2009 the visionary John Mackey wooed me away from firefighting by offering me a platform to take helping people and saving lives to a whole new level, and I am forever grateful. These last seven years have been some of the most fulfilling and growth-expanding years of my life. I also want to thank the 1,000-plus team members who have come to an Engine 2 Seven-Day Rescue program. And I want to directly thank John Mackey, Walter Robb, Betsy Foster, and Patricia Petty for their support of the immersion programs. I have learned so much from all of you.

There are many other people I wish to thank. These include:

- Claire Osborn, a reporter with the *Austin American-Statesman*, for setting this Engine 2 world in motion in 2005 by writing the article "Tofu Outmuscles Red Meat at Firehouse."
- Inkwell Management and my brilliant literary agent, Richard Pine, for pushing me to write a third book.
- Grand Central Publishing and Jamie Raab; Matthew Ballast; Nick Small; Julie Paulauski; my editor, Sarah Pelz; and Jon Contino for his brilliant work with the cover design for this book! Thank you all for staying by my side and helping us share this important message.
- The Engine 2 team members who have helped produce Seven-Day Rescue programs from Austin, Texas, to the Big Island of Hawaii and to Sedona, Arizona; Adam Reiser, who has been my dynamic events partner since we began this journey in 2010; Jillian Gibson, one of the hardest-working operation managers ever; Dani Little, the Engine 2 plant-nutritionist and dietician who has been with me at Whole Foods through it all; Nathan

and Kristin Turner, great friends and cutting-edge fitness trainers (as well as Porangui impersonators); Adam Sud, a new friend, one hell of a motivational speaker, and one of the most amazing life turnarounds I've ever seen; Brenda Reed, a force of kindness and our amazing head chef in the kitchen; Dr. Linda Carney and her husband, Sean Carney, our first medical directors; Dr. Stuart Seale, our second medical director; and Dr. Don Forrester, our third medical director and speaker.

- The amazing speakers we have had over the years who have not only taught the participants but have also taught me. These include: Jeff Novick, a mighty force with his knowledge, talks, and acts of strength; Doug Lisle, the psychologist who helps keep all of us sane; Michael Klaper, a kind and caring physician; T. Colin Campbell and his push for a whole-food, plant-based diet; John Robbins, for sharing his light; Pam Popper, for her wealth of knowledge and constant calm; Dr. Garth Davis, for jumping into the plant-strong arena and teaching weight-loss patients about the power of plants; and Dr. Mladen Golubic, for stepping in and saving the day when we needed it.

- Ami Mackey, the Engine 2 creative content curator, for always being at the ready to do anything and everything, including recipe development, photography, food lists, copy, analytics, or food coaching.

- Char Nolan, the E2 connector, for her grace, confidence, and her staying power with Engine 2 and the Esselstyn family.

- Rick Kent, aka "Brother Love," for his friendship and photography skills.

- Anne Stevenson, for her muffins and for her amazing graphic design work.

- Mike Schall, for his unwavering support and loyalty with Engine 2 and with our friendship.

- Mike McKeon, for his steady hand and level head with all things surrounding the Engine 2 Plant-Strong food line.

- The Nelson family, for their love and support: Jeff, Sabrina, Will, and the twins, Nina and Randa.

- Brian Hart, for his enthusiasm and keen instincts as he enters the plant-strong world.

- Karen Flaherty, for being not only a rock star but a rock, for Engine 2 and for Jill and me.
- Eleanor Rimmerman, for testing, reading, and editing so many recipes.
- Wade Clark, for his photography and videography skills.
- Laurie Kortowitch, who was sent to me from the plant-strong heavens and has now taken on the role of the Engine 2 program coordinator. She is an absolute diamond! Laurie was the force behind organizing the two pilot studies for this book, Hyland Software and the City of North Ridgeville.

I am also very grateful to the organizations and people associated with the pilot studies for this book. These include Plant-Based Cleveland's Amy Wing, Greg Wing, and Marianne Antonelli, for their phenomenal support in implementing the Hyland Software and North Ridgeville pilot studies; the entire North Ridgeville Heart and Sole Collaborate, including the determined Erin Murphy, and also Rita Price, Kevin Fougerousse, Meredith Brescilli, and Don Schiffbauer, who found us the supplies we needed to screen our North Ridgeville participants. A special shout-out goes to the City of North Ridgeville's open-minded mayor, David Gillock. I also want to thank the Lorain County Metroparks and Jim Ziemnik and Jennifer Bracken for the use of their beautiful facility, as well as the Lorain County General Health District; United Way of Greater Lorain County and Bill Harper; Hyland Software, a company bursting with innovation and blazing a trail of plant-strong wellness—and specifically Miguel Zubizarreta, Tiffany Scherer, Liz Simon, Jackie McNamara, Brenda Kirk, and Rob Hawkins; Pioneer Ridge by Del Webb, for their unbridled support and commitment to this project; and the City of Mesquite, Texas, employees and their health coordinator, Elizabeth Jones, for hosting and supporting the first Seven-Day Rescue pilot in July 2015.

A very big thank-you goes out to my parents, Ann and Essy, who have been the most supportive superhero parents a kid could ever dream up. They have been so instrumental in Engine 2's success, whether it's been the Seven-Day Rescue programs, the weekend events, or the books, and they have witnessed my transformation from a firefighter to a plant-strong eating advocate. It's been a dream to be able to team up with them and share this message of health and hope.

Likewise, I want to give a Texas-size thank-you to my sister, Jane Esselstyn, for spearheading part 2 of this book and for her passion for all things Engine 2 and plant-strong. There is nothing that Jane hasn't done at our Seven-Day Rescue programs, including planning the menus, speaking, food demos, dancing, leading hikes, and getting just about everyone to break out of their shells!

Of course, I want to thank the rest of my family for all their support as well: Ted Esselstyn and Anne Bingham, Zeb Esselstyn, Polly LaBarre; Flinn, Gus, Rose, Crile, "Little" Zeb, Bainon, Georgie, and my aunt Susie Crile.

Finally, thank you, Nick Bromley, for your writing skills, research, and humor. And, of course, thank you, Gene Stone, my writing partner— for hanging in there with me for our third book, for your patience, for teaching me to stick to my instincts, for pushing me when appropriate, and for our warm and thoughtful friendship over the last eight incredible years.

Most of all, I want to thank my loving and steadfast wife, Jill, my energetic son, Kole, my insightful daughter Sophie, and my indefatigable daughter, Hope. You all keep me grounded and brimming over with light and love. I love you all to the moon and back. Twice! Three times!

Index

About the Author

RIP ESSELSTYN was born in upstate New York, raised in Cleveland, Ohio, and attended the University of Texas at Austin, where he was a three-time All-American swimmer and majored in speech communications. After graduation Rip spent a decade as one of the world's premier triathletes. He then joined the Austin Fire Department where he introduced his passion for a whole-food, plant-based diet to Austin's Engine 2 Firehouse in order to rescue a firefighting brother's health. To document his success, he wrote the national best-selling book *The Engine 2 Diet*, which shows the irrefutable connection between a plant-based diet and good health. His second book, *Plant-Strong*, became a #1 *New York Times* best seller.

Seven years ago, Rip left his job as a firefighter to team up with Whole Foods Market as one of their Healthy Eating Partners to raise awareness for team members, customers, and communities about the benefits of eating a whole-food, plant-strong diet. He has appeared on numerous national television shows, including the *Today* show, *CBS This Morning*, *Good Morning America*, and the *Dr. Oz Show*.

Rip is married to Jill Kolasinski and they have three children, Kole, Sophie, and Hope. They live in Austin, Texas.